Moving Beyond

A.D.D. A.D.H.D.

An Effective, All Natural, Holistic, Mind-Body Approach

Second Edition

Transpersonal Publishing

All of the publisher's titles, imprints, and distributed lines are
available at special quantity discounts for bulk purchases for sales
promotions, premiums, fund-raising, and educational or institutional
use. Special book excerpts or customized printings can also be
created to fit specific needs. For details, contact the publisher:

Transpersonal Publishing, div. AHU, LLC
P.O. Box 7220, Kill Devil Hills, NC 27948
800-296-MIND

Wholesale—
www.TranspersonalPublishing.com or
orders@holistictree.com, or
distributed by SCB Distributors
and available through all major wholesalers

Retail—
www.Holistictree.com/store or (800) 296-MIND

Library of Congress Control Number (LCCN): 2007940248

To Brian, with much love. Always my inspiration, you helped me stretch beyond my reach.

Rita Kirsch Debroitner

For all parents, children, and adults who are willing to start with themselves. Enjoy your well-earned freedom!

Avery Hart

Rita Kirsch Debroitner CSW-R, PhD, is a Holistic Psychotherapist. Dr. Kirsch is creator and founder of the Rhinecliff Non-drug ADD/ADHD Program. She is also author of: *There's Nothing Wrong With You, Adam* and *Please Don't Eat The Crayons Harry*. Both books give practical information for moving beyond ADD/ADHD. She has a practice in Rhinecliff, NY, and Boerum Hill, Brooklyn, where Harry and Tai, a Bichon and yellow lab, are pet therapists who help others with moving beyond.

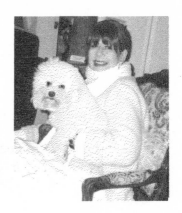

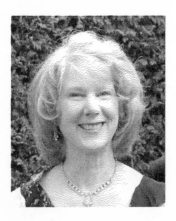

Avery Hart is an award-winning childrens book author and practicing psychotherapist. Her other books include: *Kids Make Music, Kids Garden, Pyramids!, Who Really Discovered America?,* and *Boredom Busters*. Avery received a BA from Penn State University, MA from New York University, MSW from Yeshiva University, and PhD from Clayton College of Natural Health.

Swimming against an icy torrent . . .
Navigating through a cave of poisonous fog . . .
Taking aim, and shooting faster than the enemy . . .

If you are involved with A.D.D./A.D.H.D. as an adult or parent of an A.D.D./A.D.H.D.-identified child, your life has more in common with the hero or heroine of an action movie than you might realize—with a couple of unsettling differences.

The movie hero knows that the adventure will end in a matter of hours, with victory assured. For the person struggling with the symptoms of A.D.D./A.D.H.D., however, the action continues day after day, year after year; the outcome is far from certain and fraught with danger.

If you have felt hopeless, helpless, fatigued, and discouraged, welcome to the A.D.D./A.D.H.D. club. If you wish to trade in those discouraged feelings for a different experience—one of enhanced ability to grapple with the disorder and ultimately triumph over it—place your hand on your heart right now, because that is the place where true and lasting transformation can begin.

Contents

Foreword

The book in your hands is timely and sorely needed. No threat to our future is as real, immediate, and calamitous as the internal and external biologic and emotional health hazards that we and our children face day to day. Attention deficit and related disorders are claiming new victims at an alarming rate. The individuals involved, both children and adults, are living on metabolic and emotional roller coasters, suffering from wild mood swings, experiencing internal distress, and creating havoc with their impulsive behavior.

When I began my study of medicine nearly four decades ago, a medical student could spend weeks in a pediatric clinic without encountering one child disabled by attention deficit disorder, learning disabilities, autism, or any related disorder. Now hardly a day passes when I do not hear a heartrending description by a mother agonizing over her child's difficulties in living. Adults, too—particularly young adults—report a similar torment about their inability to build their lives in an organized fashion. What is the answer to this suffering?

The *Journal of the American Medical Association* reports that the number of children diagnosed with A.D.D. consistently doubled every four to seven years, from 1971 to 1987, to the point that in a typical American city approximately 6% of children are receiving psychotropic medication.

A consistent doubling of the rate of medication treatment! Where did this frightening epidemic come from? Is it a new viral affliction that is causing the neuronal misfiring? Is the condition caused by a new bacterium or mutated yeast, or perhaps a parasite imported to the United States and other western nations?

Is the culprit an obscure pesticide or a dragon unleashed by synthetic chemistry? What exactly is triggering these trigger-happy neurotransmitters?

Have the genes of those afflicted with symptoms of A.D.D./A.D.H.D. gone berserk?

I don't think so.

Perhaps the most compelling question of all is: *why do afflicted children and adults do well at certain times and so poorly at others*? Why don't their genes continuously and consistently cause their nerve cells to misfire? This, in my view, is the core issue.

The epidemic of attention deficit disorder cannot be understood by nineteenth-century notions of diseases and drugs. Instead, we must learn to look at the disorder as *a violation of the natural physical, mental, and energetic ecosystems*, and then teach *that* to the afflicted individuals. *Moving Beyond A.D.D./A.D.H.D.* is a giant step in this direction.

Debroitner and Hart make an impressive argument that *when the emphasis is placed on restoring the natural energy of the body, mind, and spirit, a secure sense of mental well-being will result.* They courageously underscore the differences between the prevailing medical model of the treatment of A.D.D. and its related disorders and the new emerging model of integrative medicine.

The integrative model seeks to enlighten afflicted individuals as well as all those who care for them. The authors contend that the "treatment" in the medical model is in reality mere symptom suppression, and that the answers to the problems of A.D.D. and related learning disabilities are not in pushing pills.

One of the fundamental concepts of their approach is that children will learn to know and honor themselves only when they see the adults around them doing so. Only when adults begin moving toward freedom of toxic overload on the mental, biologic, and energy levels can they free their children of this pernicious disorder. Then, in fact, they *cannot fail* to free them. Herein, as Avery Hart and Rita Kirsch Debroitner clearly and masterfully outline, is the simplicity of true healing.

I end this foreword on a positive note. This is an exciting time. Nearly each month I see scientific articles that validate one or more of the ancient healing arts or philosophies. I fully expect that the work of the authors will continue to be validated by future research. I am honored and privileged to set the stage for *Moving Beyond A.D.D./A.D.H.D.*, a book that by its merit is destined to become a classic in its field.

Majid Ali, M.D.
President and Professor of Medicine, Capital University
of Integrative Medicine, Washington, D.C.
Associate Professor of Pathology, College of Physicians
and Surgeons of Columbia University, New York
Director, Department of Pathology, Immunology, and
Laboratories, Holy Name Hospital, Teaneck, New Jersey
Fellow, Royal College of Surgeons of England
Author: *RDA: Rats, Drugs and Assumptions* and *The
Canary and Chronic Fatigue*

Acknowledgments

To all children, adults, and families who have participated in the Rhinecliff Non-Drug A.D.D./A.D.H.D. Program and who have had the courage to face what is not working and take charge of their lives, I salute you.

To my family, who provided me treasured and growing moments. To my grandmother, Fannie Debroitner, my mother, Esther Watstein, and father, William Gaber, I thank you for your devotion. To Rose, ahead of her time, and an inspiration. To Sally and Shana Hansen with lots of love.

To Pamela, Sid, Brandon, and Tyler and Julian Schlomann and to Walter, Jo, David, and Sasha Schlomann, special thanks for being who you are.

To Warren Baldt, a true and steadfast friend. Thanks for all of your support and encouragement.

To Niravi Payne, M.S., founder of the Whole Person Fertility Program, friend and fellow traveler. Your support and input were very appreciated.

To all the teachers of the New York City school system with whom I worked and to those everywhere who go the extra mile and truly make a difference for our children. To those teachers who participated in the Non-Drug A.D.D./A.D.H.D. workshops, I salute you.

To Dr. Carl M. Kirsch, who helped me with my first steps.

To Dean Vigilante, former dean of the Social Work School at Adelphi University. Thank you for believing in me; it is truly appreciated.

To Mary Walker, M.S., for encouraging me to put my work into print.

To Gurudev, whose teachings and truth will always have an impact.

To Susan Cohen, our agent. I acknowledge your part in helping to get this project into print.

Rita Kirsch Debroitner, R.C.S.W., Ph.D.

I wish to thank Dr. Renee Schlesinger, Dr. Irving Levitz, and Norman Tokayer, outstanding teachers of Yeshiva University, and Drs. Brian Sweeney and Allan Dolber of the Fifth Avenue Center for Psychotherapy, each of whom convey with depth and clarity the process by which people can learn to locate and free their inner, authentic selves. I am also very grateful to Linda Friedricks, a dedicated clinician and caring friend who first brought my attention to the problems of A.D.D./A.D.H.D. families and inspired my search for medication-free solutions. My supportive and insightful colleagues at the Fifth Avenue Center for Psychotherapy, Larry Klein, Batya Zahmir, Laura Guastini, Lynn Schultz, Tina La Greca, and Dick Wasserman, are owed thanks, too. Each has significantly contributed to my growth and enhanced my ability to understand the process that allows people to move forward with purpose.

Additional thanks go to Dr. Joseph Gallagher, for expanding my understanding and pointing the way to appropriate research, and Drs. Joseph Trachtman and Gary Null, for sharing their expertise in treating A.D.D./A.D.H.D. without medication. I am also grateful to Victoria LaFortune, Susan Cohen, Amanda George, and Sandra Marks Gallagher for their loyal friendship and enduring faith in my abilities; my niece, Debra Wagner Walsh, M.S.W., whose love of children is both inspiring and informed. I thank Andrea Rudolph, M.S.W., for her collegial friendship; Irene Brino Wagner and Phyllis Segal, M.S.W., for their earthly wisdom; and Robert

C. Wagner and Maria Avitable, for their love and inspiration across the big divide.

Last on the list, but first in my life, thanks to Paul Mantell for his enduring love in marriage, and Clayton and Matthew Mantell, the vibrant sons who have deepened my appreciation of the joy that comes with being alive.

Avery Hart, M.S.W., M.A., C.H.T.

We both wish to thank our editor, Susan Schwartz, for her enthusiasm and support. Special thanks to Julia Anderson and Maureen Musker, for being available and helpful, and to the others at Contemporary Books who have helped make this book and work a reality. And large appreciation goes to Eleanor Ryder and the Northern Dutchess County Medical Center administrative staff for generously allowing us the use of their research facilities.

Second Edition Preface

Time has wings! It's been almost ten years since the first edition of Moving Beyond ADD/ADHD: An Effective, Holistic, Mind-Body Approach was published. Since then we have been heartened by the response of readers, and the positive results they've reported to us. In our private practices, we've continued to be involved with families, children, and adults who, with guidance and encouragement, were able to develop the kind of new and improved, present-moment consciousness that moved them beyond the symptoms of Attention Deficits-with no nasty side effects, either. Freed of Attention Deficit symptoms, these families can now spend their time and energy enjoying each other, exploring life, and developing their potential.

Our theory is simple enough: A person of any age who is centered and grounded will not have Attention Deficits. Therefore, when a person invests time and energy learning to become centered and grounded - in charge of their energy, internally balanced, and presto - the psychiatric disorder disappears! In its place is a living, breathing human being who is capable of organizing his or her energy and meeting life's inevitable challenges as they occur. The means for creating this kind of positive change are all contained within the pages of this book.

For ADD/ADHD symptomatic children, our approach starts with parents learning to become centered and grounded within themselves. Once parents learn to live their own balanced, empowered lives, the entire family dynamic automatically begins to shift. The result is a family that works for each and every member, where each member is validated and supported, able to face challenges without falling apart. Improved effectiveness at school and work naturally follows, too, as family members take their new-found awareness and life skills and begin applying them to situations outside the home.

Contrast this drug-free approach to the pharmaceutical treatment offered for Attention Deficits, and the benefits of this book becomes even more apparent.

It's now aproximately a decade into the twenty-first century, and America's venerable FDA, the agency that is supposed to protect citizens on matters of drug safety, is in disgrace. So much bad news has been exposed about the workings of a health care system in which profitability trumps integrity - even when the health of our most vulnerable citizens, children, is at stake. During 2004, Americans learned of a rising rate of childhood suicide connected to psychiatric drugs, and worse: The very officials who were supposed to protect the public were found to have purposefully suppressed information about the dangers of several manufactured medications! In Canada, after fourteen young people died as a result of Adderall, that drug has been banned. England is encouraging clinicians to seek only drug-free approaches for ADD and ADHD.

And yet the drugging of American children continues in a pattern of unhappiness: Families are in trouble, struggling to cope with the stress of ADD/ADHD symptoms. Doctors try to relieve symptoms by prescribing drugs. And the problems of ADD/ADHD symptoms spin on, veering off this way or that in a dizzy circle of upsets. For challenging cases, new labels emerge for negative, out-of-control behavior and chaotic, foggy perspectives, such as the rise of childhood bi-polarity. Sadly, many families are unaware that safer and more effective treatment options even exist!

Drugs may mask ADD problems for a time, but it is only human beings, using their own power from within, that can overcome and cure those problems permanently. How rewarding it is to see a family move beyond ADD/ADHD - closer to each other – stronger at heart – and more effective in the world!

Yes, you can move beyond ADD/ADHD...we all can! We can move beyond a society of labels, dysfunctions, and disorders. We can move beyond looking outside of ourselves for answers - beyond negativity and worry. There's a beautiful land waiting for those who find their personal power and grapple with reality: Let's go there!

Introduction

A New Approach for a New Epidemic

Everything should be made as simple as possible, but no simpler.

Albert Einstein

You have picked up this book because you care deeply about someone identified as having A.D.D. or A.D.H.D. It may be your child, your husband, or even yourself. You may be wondering if this person really has attention deficit and, if so, what can be done about it.

You've heard about A.D.D. and A.D.H.D., but still, questions may be spinning through your brain. Is it an invisible brain disease or neurological flaw? Will Ritalin help, or will it create lasting harm? Why is this happening to you?

Every day in this nation, thousands of good people find themselves in a similar position. Attention deficit disorder, with or without hyperactivity, is the name given to a cluster of symptoms. It has swept across America, bringing upset and confusion wherever it goes. Conservative estimates are that 3 to 5% of American children have already been diagnosed with the disorder.[1] Because the majority of diagnosed children are male, some social scientists believe that 10% or more of American boys are affected.

Many of the parents of these children, in desperation, seek help in the form of a prescription: for Ritalin, Cylert, Clonodine, or other medications. But a nagging doubt often remains.

Our intention is to help you sort out your options and clarify the issues that underlie A.D.D./A.D.H.D., so that you will have a broader understanding of the disorder. We don't have all the answers—nobody does—but we *can* light the way by offering you an approach to the disorder that is both unique and effective.

We know that there is a solution to the problem of A.D.D./A.D.H.D. because we've seen it. We've experienced the transformation of children, adults, and families who have had the courage to face the disorder, starting with themselves, and take the necessary actions to eliminate it from their lives. We've seen parents reclaim their power, and children reclaim their potential, triumphing over the disorder that had previously caused so much misery in their family lives.

All those who have moved beyond A.D.D./A.D.H.D. started where you may be today: in a state of confusion and frustration, tired of wrestling with a difficult foe, and on the edge of hopelessness as they read that many experts believe the disorder can never be cured, only managed. Many parents and spouses whose lives are affected by A.D.D./A.D.H.D. are anxious—understandably so—about the future of their loved one who carries the symptoms.

If you are in a helping profession, as a primary care physician, therapist, or teacher, reading this book to expand your understanding of A.D.D./A.D.H.D., you too may wonder if it's possible for people to have a full and complete restoration to health.

Well, it is.

A.D.D./A.D.H.D. does *not* have to be a chronic condition.

A Holistic Approach

Every day with A.D.D./A.D.H.D., routine events such as getting dressed, mealtimes, and homework become an exercise in discord and teeth-gritting frustration for parents, and feelings of failure and low self-esteem for kids. The same negative feelings follow adult A.D.D./A.D.H.D. sufferers throughout the day.

A.D.D./A.D.H.D. kids fidget, dawdle, and shriek, acting out their negative, disconnected emotions. They create an upside-down world for their caregivers. Adults carrying the symptoms have usually learned to mask their difficulties somewhat, but under the surface of their lives, they are living with the same restless negativity and feelings of alienation and disconnection.

Fortunately, there are ways to assist yourself, as the parent of an A.D.D./A.D.H.D. child, or as an adult who carries the symptoms. Through self-empowerment, anyone whose life is affected by attention deficits and impulsivity can become stronger than the disorder itself.

Moving Beyond A.D.D./A.D.H.D. will provide you with a holistic understanding of the disorder, and give you cohesive strategies and concrete tools to combat it. When this understanding is put into action, you will find yourself and your loved one gradually shifting from a helpless, reactive existence to an empowered and secure one. *Our holistic approach offers a new perspective—one of positive, self-sustaining action that enables A.D.D./A.D.H.D.-diagnosed people and their loved ones to shift away from their negative symptoms, effectively freeing themselves of the disorder.*

Every aspect of living is explored from this perspective, from internal attitudes to external postures; from diet and lifestyle choices to care of the brain. We also focus on the often overlooked but vital understanding of how A.D.D./A.D.H.D. people use (or misuse) their senses to take in signals and information from the world around them. This sensory information will help readers identify problem areas, so they can begin to correct them.

Another important theme of this book is movement and the use of the body. We strongly believe that the way one moves, shapes, or forms one's body is *both a symbolic and real communication about the person's inner state of being*, and as such can offer important clues about how to affect positive change. This work, psychostructural dynamics (PSD), was developed by coauther Rita Kirsch Debroitner, and is described below.

We believe that approaching the disorder from a mind-body and energy perspective makes perfect sense, because the A.D.D./A.D.H.D. mind–body and energy are out of sync with each other. This lack of inner accord creates an ongoing state of anxiety and confusion. As the mind, body, and energy are all involved in the development of the disorder, these levels need to be aligned and work harmoniously for recovery to occur.

For parents and others concerned about the potentially harmful physical and emotional effects of psychopharmaceutical drugs, relevant information is presented, including information about alternative substances that may be helpful in restoring biochemical balance.

The good news is there are simple but proven strategies and techniques that improve the overall functioning of the body and brain, emotions, senses, self-connection, and self-creativity, which ultimately eliminate A.D.D./A.D.H.D. symptoms. In each case, we have strived to boil complex issues and information down to their most useful form.

The connection between self-esteem and self-mastery is also explored, drawing on Avery Hart's experience as a psychoanalyst, children's author, and educator.

The latter chapters of the book describe in broad terms the landscape that lies beyond A.D.D./A.D.H.D., touching on the emergence of the secure self into the larger world of one's special abilities and interests, friendships, connection to nature, and place in the universe. The A.D.D.-free individual is one who is connected and comfortable as an individual on social and spiritual levels.

We think of *Moving Beyond A.D.D./A.D.H.D.* as an interactive book and hope that you will use it this way. Reading about ideas is useful, but directly experiencing them is far more powerful. Our work with those who have recovered from A.D.D./A.D.H.D. has taught us that *true and lasting changes of heart, mind, and body ultimately come from taking responsibility for one's experience, and putting new ideas into everyday action until they become second nature.*

How This Book Came to Be Written

As a student of self-psychology, a treatment theory that emphasizes the need for a secure inner self, I (Avery) had witnessed remarkable progress in clients who learned to identify their authentic needs and consciously organize their life experiences. Adding cognitive and behavioral exercises and techniques based in clinical hypnosis, such as creative visualization and deep relaxation, seemed to hasten and increase positive change in my clients, freeing the natural development of the inner self. I became convinced, through my experiences and those of others in our field, that self-cohesion, self-security, and the restoration of inner vitality were key factors to A.D.D. recovery for children as well as adults.

My observations about the lifestyle choices of A.D.D. clients and long interest in nutrition and media awareness were also significant, arousing my curiousity about the impact of routinized TV, diet, and lifestyle factors on the development of A.D.D.

In 1995 I set off on an adventure to identify the causes, as well as the most effective nonpharmaceutical solutions, to attention deficit problems and present them to the public. This exploration eventually led me to Rita's door, and to our collaboration on this book.

I (Rita) had been working with A.D.D. clients since 1987 using a holistic, drug-free approach, and had been planning to write a book about my discoveries and experiences. When Avery contacted me, it seemed natural for us to collaborate on a definitive book that would help children, parents, teachers, and adults to move beyond A.D.D. without medication.

The system I created, psychostructural dynamics (PSD), stresses factors such as the relationship to one's self as the primary power in one's life, body alignment, mind–body connection, as well as the capacity to heal and live in tune with one's natural state of being. The theories and techniques of PSD have been adapted and incorporated in my Rhinecliff Non-Drug A.D.D./A.D.H.D. Program. In centers located in Rhinecliff, Manhattan, and Brooklyn Heights, New York, hundreds of children and adults have successfully moved beyond A.D.D. The tools and techniques of this program are included in our book, illustrated by stories of the people who have learned to tune into themselves and live more effectively, experiencing greater freedom and joy.

Together, during the preparation of *Moving Beyond A.D.D./A.D.H.D.*, we have searched for useful information from other countries, where drugs are rarely prescribed to children. International studies of A.D.D./A.D.H.D. are not readily available to most Americans and we believe our readers deserve to know about them.

Our collaboration has been a productive and positive experience, allowing both of us to grow as we enhanced and refined our understanding of what it takes to move beyond A.D.D.

There are no instant magic solutions to the problem of attention deficits, of course. But based on the results attained at the Centers and in our private practices, we can confidently assure you that our comprehensive, holistic approach makes progress against the disorder, steady and sure. If you are looking to eliminate the negativity of A.D.D./A.D.H.D. from your life, you have come to the right place and opened the right book.

The Miracle Within

In our work, we've seen, time and again, the transformation of A.D.D./A.D.H.D.-diagnosed people as they become more grounded, connected, and in touch with themselves on a mental, physical, and energy level. When that happens, negative symptoms such as acting out and low self-esteem fall away. Nothing allows a person's authentic self-esteem to rise more than mastery of self, and nothing dissolves negative behavior better than true self-respect. Pointing the way to self-empowerment for the diagnosed person is the heart and soul of our process.

Once an A.D.D./A.D.H.D. person experiences him- or herself as capable, cooperative, positive, and in control on a body, mind, and energy level, the results are nothing less than astounding. An internal transformation takes place, affecting the unseen self, deep within, as well as the person's use of his or her eyes, ears, heart, and mind. The internal transformation concurs with the emotional, psychological, and physical release from A.D.D./A.D.H.D.

Freed of the negative symptoms, people can stand strong and learn to know themselves, while experiencing feelings of calm, true wholeness. They have now moved into the center of their own experience and consequently proceed from balance, no longer prey to every passing distraction and internal impulse.

These miraculous outcomes are not the result of a miracle from on high—they're the result of a miracle *within*, a miracle of self-healing and self-empowerment that lies within anyone's grasp.

No Guilt, No Blame

Deep inside, if you are an adult suffering from A.D.D., or the parent of an A.D.D/A.D.H.D. child, you may sometimes feel inadequate or be burdened with intolerable feelings of self-blame. Parents of attention deficit-diagnosed children often worry that they have somehow caused the disorder in their children. Adults whose lives are caught in the mire of impulsivity and disorder may judge themselves harshly for being the way they are.

Guilt, blame, fault, shame—these concepts have no place in the healing process we offer within these pages. To the extent that they are operative, even if locked up and kept out of conscious awareness, the person struggling with the effects of the disorder remains frozen and stuck in a negative, reactive state. Guilt, blame, fault, and shame affect everyone and create the breeding ground for one of A.D.D./A.D.H.D.'s hallmark symptoms: low self-esteem.

Low self-esteem is one of the disorder's constant companions. So strong is it that it seems to affect everyone who regularly interacts with the person, as if pulling others into the negative vortex of A.D.D. symptomology, where out-of-control feelings tumble and spin with lack of perspective. *The pain of feeling not good enough becomes the basis of emotional suffering for child, parent, teacher, caregiver, or self.* This feeling of inadequacy lurks in the shadow of all negative behavior and experience, blocking the path to new possibilities or positive action.

We would like to call the essentially negative concepts of guilt, blame, fault, and shame out of the shadows so that they can be seen for what they are: *thieves.* For what this ugly foursome really does is rob us of precious *energy*—energy that can otherwise be channeled into taking positive action against the disorder.

By letting go of blame and guilt, you take the first step toward turning your topsy-turvy A.D.D. world right-side up again and restoring peace, positive energy, and even joy to your family life.

Have You Been Here?

From the holistic perspective, every human being has the right and capacity to create a fulfilling life in which the individual's authentic self can safely emerge and develop. This natural state of being, at the core of every self, is every individual's birthright; it is the energy that drives the unlimited potential of an individual to develop, grow, and heal. In A.D.D./A.D.H.D., the process of self-development can seem to be stalled, creating situations like these:

- The teacher called again today to complain about your child. You know your child is bright, but the teacher reports that he's disruptive and doesn't listen. It's clear that she wants him taken to a doctor and tested for A.D.H.D.

- Your daughter lost her knapsack again, for the fourth time this year. She's so disorganized! Getting her ready for school is a major effort that leaves you exhausted by 9 A.M. She seems to try hard. . . . Maybe she has a real problem. . . .

- Your son kicked you in the shin when a friend was visiting, and you felt humiliated and embarrassed. Your friend seemed to feel sorry for you. She asked if you were going to get some help. You know she thinks he has A.D.D.

- When it was time to leave the toy store, your child threw a major tantrum. He plunked himself down in the aisle, yelling and calling you cheap. His tantrums are all too frequent. Maybe there really is something wrong with him. Maybe he has A.D.H.D.

- You were making dinner when your child burst into the kitchen and opened the fridge. You asked him to wait, but he said he couldn't. To make it worse, he hit his younger sister for no apparent reason. Now she's crying, and he's yelling, and the dinner you planned has been ruined. When you tell your mother about it that night on the phone, she asks, "What's wrong with that kid?"

• Other children seem to play without much supervision, but not your child. Even though he's eight years old, he's constantly getting into trouble the minute you leave him alone. He just squirted the neighbor's dog with a hose for the third time this week. Now your neighbor is fuming. "That kid of yours is not normal!"

You Are Not Alone

When A.D.D./A.D.H.D. is a factor in a person's life, the individual often feels overwhelmed, burdened, and burned out. He or she also may feel terribly alone, but nothing could be further from the truth. Attention deficit has become the fastest growing diagnosis of children and adolescents in the United States, and it is rapidly increasing in adults.[2] Other developed nations, particularly those involved in the global economy, show a rise as well, though not as dramatic.[3]

It's intriguing to consider why A.D.D. is a phenomenon of western nations. Many reputable experts believe that the consumption of highly processed, artificial foods and internal food allergies are a factor. This possibility will be discussed in Chapter 8. Some believe that environmental toxins and pollutants are implicated in the development of the disorder. This idea, too, appears to have some validity for A.D.H.D. based on animal studies, but it has yet to be definitively proven for human beings.[4]

On the other hand, the emergence of routinized TV viewing is a little-publicized but significant and *proven* cause of hyperactivity.[5] Understanding the effect of commercial TV and other lifestyle choices is important to our understanding of the disorder and will be explored later in this book.

The search for root causes on which we have embarked grew out of a sense of empathy with our clients and the need to understand their suffering. When these ordinary, extraordinary people first entered treatment, they were caught between desperation and hope. But they had the courage to face themselves, and hone their self-awareness from moment to moment, gradually triumphing over the disorder. The experiences of these individuals are the basis of our inspiration for writing this book, and they have generously allowed us to use their stories to illuminate the confounding factors of A.D.D./A.D.H.D.

If you have been living with the disorder, you will surely recognize yourself in their stories. Our hope is that this recognition will propel you into action—internal action—so that you too will be freed to release yourself from the grip of A.D.D./A.D.H.D.

"But wait," you may say, "isn't A.D.D. a brain disease or neurological impairment?" Many intelligent, educated people are under the mistaken impression that attention deficit disorder is caused by a malfunction or problem in the brain or central nervous system. The truth is that *there is little or no scientific evidence to support this belief.* Before the term "attention deficit" came into use, children with A.D.D./A.D.H.D. symptoms were referred to as "brain injured," or said to have "minimal brain damage or dysfunction." It is perplexing to laypeople that medical professionals would use such terms when no evidence of any injury, damage, or organic dysfunction exists. Nevertheless, that is exactly what happened.[6]

In the 1930s doctors created the scientific-sounding term "brain injured" to describe impulsive, out-of-control children. This label was probably perceived as an improvement over previous descriptors such as "monstrous," "bad," or "bratty."

There was just one problem—no brain injury was ever discovered to justify the use of the term.

By the 1960s, the medical profession jettisoned the "brain injured" label, replacing it instead with "minimal brain damage" and "minimal brain dysfunction." These terms, too, were scientifically inaccurate, however, and ultimately insupportable.

In 1980 when a Canadian social scientist coined the term "attention deficits," mental health and medical professionals quickly adopted it for use. Today, further confusion arises from the use of the term *neurological*. Few people are told that this scientific-sounding word is often used by doctors as a synonym for psychological or emotional-based. Similarly, the word "genetic" is sometimes used inaccurately to imply a physical base for a problem because all other explanations have failed.

In the service of the idea that symptoms of A.D.D./A.D.H.D. must have a physical cause, researchers have searched for decades to find a specific flaw that would explain the growing epidemic of dysfunctional behavior in young people. Despite this effort, *no definitive or consistent physical neurological impairment has ever been determined. That is the reason no standard test for A.D.D./A.D.H.D. exists.*

Weird Science

Scientifically speaking, the terms A.D.D. and A.D.H.D. do not refer to a specific disease—instead they are labels for a cluster of symptoms. Saying that someone "has" A.D.D. is like saying a person has R.N.D., Runny Nose Disorder.

Traditional science depends on the study of specific variables or factors. But in the case of attention deficit, studying variables is all but impossible, since the definition of symptoms depends on the subjective opinion of observers.

Many studies indicate that neither parents, teachers, doctors, social workers, nor psychologists can agree about A.D.D./ A.D.H.D. symptoms when observing human behavior in action.[7] One man's hyperactivity is another man's exuberance. What is impulsive to one person can be spontaneous to another. Inattentiveness can seem the normal and natural reaction to certain circumstances to one person, and inappropriate to someone else in similar circumstances.

It's important to keep in mind that psychiatric diagnoses tend to reflect social concerns as well as hard science. For example, homosexuality was defined as a mental health disorder in the official diagnostic and statistical manual of the American Psychiatric Association, until 1980, when the diagnosis could no longer be justified. As recently as 1994, a psychiatric diagnosis of self-defeating personality disorder appeared in this manual. But when the new disorder was strongly criticized by groups who feared it would be used against women, it was quietly dropped.

We believe that nonprofessionals need to understand the distinction between old-fashioned laboratory medical research and new-fashioned psychiatric and social research. It's important to keep psychiatric diagnoses in perspective. Creating diagnostic guidelines and behavioral diagnoses is simply how physicians and mental health professionals organize the real problems that real people are having, so they can talk about them in a coherent way.

Changing Brains and the Emperor's New Genes

The many studies searching for a biological source of A.D.D./ A.D.H.D. have failed to establish a definitive physiological neurological or genetic cause of the disorder. One study initially showed a problem with glucose processing in the brains of A.D.H.D.-diagnosed adults, but the results have never been duplicated, despite numerous attempts.[8]

Some researchers are currently focusing on the possibility of neurotransmitter dysfunction as the cause of A.D.D./A.D.H.D. This theory, too, remains unproven. Another provocative study, also never replicated, points to a possibility that the corpus collosum, the part of the brain that links the right and left hemispheres, is slightly smaller in hyperactive individuals.[9] Coincidently, this book includes information about activities that are known to promote better balance between the hemispheres because these activities are harmonious to the principles and ideas we hold about the process of moving beyond A.D.D./A.D.H.D.

The larger truth here is that *the human brain is unlike any other organ in the body because its internal structure is always changing and developing as a result of experience.* For instance, the corpus collosum tends to be slightly larger in children who study music.[10]

Human beings' internal chemistry is sensitive to many factors—magnetic and electrical fields, nutrition, information from the senses, phases of the moon, exercise, light, thoughts and emotions, sleep patterns, breathing patterns, and even psychotherapy.[11] New evidence indicates that brain chemistry may even be affected by the thoughts and feelings of others in our environment. We are only at the dawn of mind-body understanding, with much to discover.

A picture of brain activity such as a position-emission tomography, or PET scan, that is taken when a person is in a relaxed state, for instance, will differ from the image of the same brain when the person is under stress.[12]

Those who are invested in the idea that A.D.D./A.D.H.D. is an invisible brain disease may be longing for a neat label or simple explanation of something that is in fact difficult to understand, complex, and multidimensional. Ironically, believing that A.D.D./A.D.H.D. has a concrete physical cause based in the brain brings a sense of relief to many people who long for an explanation for all that they have been through.

Wanting to believe that the disorder is primarily physically based and can be corrected by a substance is an all too human mistake. People who cling to this belief will even disregard what their common sense tells them. Parents often raise the same question: Why can my child focus and pay attention when he has something interesting to do? Why does my child function well in a one-on-one situation, but not in a group?

Why, indeed?

It follows that if the causes of the problems were rooted in brain or neurological malfunctions, they would be in effect at all times.

Similarly, if the disorder were truly a genetic or neurological impairment as some people believe, how can we explain its prevalence among firstborn, or first-adopted boys?[13] It's difficult to conceive that birth order could be a factor in a genetic or neurological impairment.

We believe that the national obsession with genetics to help explain social or psychological dysfunction has met its limits in A.D.D./A.D.H.D. (and other behavioral disorders). Strengthening our conviction are recent animal studies that found that brain chemicals and *genes themselves are altered by experience.*[14]

It follows, then, that to alter the biology of A.D.D./A.D.H.D. we must alter the everyday human experiences of the individuals suffering from its symptoms.

Is A.D.D./A.D.H.D. Inherited?

Although no large-scale studies have been undertaken to date, strong indications are that A.D.D./A.D.H.D. runs in families, with estimates of the rates of the disorder as high as 43% among the children of adult sufferers.[15] While some take this as evidence that attention deficit disorder has genetic root causes, we believe that the inheritance factor is more likely related to *learned behaviors.*

Hot tempers and shyness also run in families. Should we use our valuable energies and resources searching for the genetic defects of those problem behaviors as well? Isn't it wiser to confront the problems of A.D.D./A.D.H.D. behaviors and feelings in the here and now, where they truly exist and have an impact on the quality of life?

Learned behaviors can be unlearned—and A.D.D./A.D.H.D. does not have to be a permanent feature in any family's life.

A Multifaceted Problem

We believe that the *holistic model* far more accurately reflects the true nature of the disorder. A.D.D./A.D.H.D. is not a dysfunction of the central nervous system, but it *is* a condition of *imbalance,* or *disharmony,* on a dynamic, mind–body level. These imbalances have physical counterparts—in body alignment, in the use of the body, in the ability to integrate the senses, and in brain wave and biochemical functioning.

Whatever its causes, A.D.D. is a *departure from the natural core*—that grounded, centered level of being that is our human birthright.

In our professional practice, we have found that the physical aspects of A.D.D./A.D.H.D. are connected to *an inability to be at the center of one's own experience.* People with attention deficit tend to be speeded up, alienated from themselves and their experience at the most fundamental level of being. They are therefore unable to use their energy properly and function effectively.

Uncentered, they cannot "make sense" of what their senses are telling them. This, in turn, can lead to social problems that make for excess frustration in living.

Treating A.D.D./A.D.H.D. as a whole system makes sense, for we are far more than the sum of our parts—be they biological, physical, emotional, or social.

To be fully healthy, we must be *whole.*

Official Criteria

The following lists comprise the symptoms of attention deficit disorder and attention deficit disorder with hyperactivity, according to the American Psychiatric Association. Their official manual, the DSM *(Diagnostic and Statistical Manual)*, is used by insurance companies, school personnel, and mental health clinicians. Because A.D.D. and A.D.H.D. are listed as pediatric diagnoses, in adults the disorder is termed A.D.D. with or without hyperactivity residual type.

Symptoms of A.D.D. (Attention Deficit Disorder Without Hyperactivity)

Six or more of the following symptoms of inattention have persisted for at least six months to a degree that is inconsistent with the developmental level.

1. Often fails to give close attention to details; makes careless mistakes in school or other activities

2. Often has difficulty sustaining attention in tasks or play activities

3. Often does not seem to listen when spoken to directly

4. Often does not follow through on instructions and fails to finish chores or duties

5. Often has difficulty organizing tasks and activities

6. Often avoids, dislikes, or is reluctant to engage in tasks that require sustained mental effort

7. Often loses things necessary for tasks or activities

8. Is often easily distracted

9. Is often forgetful in daily activities

Symptoms of A.D.H.D.
(Attention Deficit Disorder with Hyperactivity)

Six (or more) of the following symptoms of *hyperactivity-impulsivity* have persisted for at least six months to a degree that is not consistent with the developmental level.

Hyperactivity:

1. Often fidgets with hands or feet or squirms in seat

2. Often leaves seat in classroom or other setting where sitting is required

3. Often runs about or climbs in situations in which it is inappropriate

4. Has difficulty playing or engaging in quiet leisure-time activities

5. Is often "on the go" or acts as if "driven by a motor"

6. Often talks excessively

Impulsivity

7. Often blurts out answers before question has been completed

8. Has difficulty awaiting turn

9. Often interrupts or intrudes on others (butts into conversations or games)

The Underdiagnosed, Overdiagnosed, Misdiagnosed Diagnosis

We have learned that the more you review the literature about A.D.D./A.D.H.D., the more confused you may become. Some experts claim that in thousands of children—mostly girls— A.D.D. is *under*diagnosed. They say that "the inattentive symptoms of children who are not hyperactive frequently don't call attention to themselves." These experts claim that many people who are unable to organize themselves or control their impulses are not receiving the help they need. Other experts claim that the disorder is *over*diagnosed and that millions of American children are being unnecessarily labeled as having symptoms that in fact resemble nothing more than normal immaturity.

While the over- or underdiagnosis of A.D.D. is a matter of speculation, its *mis*diagnosis is an established fact. Walter Reed Military Hospital in Washington, D.C., has conducted a thorough assessment of A.D.D./A.D.H.D.-diagnosed children who were being given medication to control their symptoms. *Approximately 50% of the children did not meet the standards outlined in the* DSM.[16]

This report and other research studies indicate that the wrongly diagnosed children may be suffering from anxiety, depression, or the aftereffects of traumatic occurrences.[17] As a society, we Americans seem reluctant to admit that our children may be depressed or anxious despite the fact that millions of adults suffer from depression, anxiety, or panic disorders.

A few cases at Walter Reed Hospital were identified as normal children of high-achieving parents who mistakenly believed that the stimulant medication often prescribed for A.D.D. improves school performance.

True Expertise

The truth is, if you are grappling with A.D.D./A.D.H.D., *you have to become your own expert*, seeking solutions from *within*. When you take charge of understanding the disorder, you become an important part of the solution.

You don't have to wait for the experts to agree. Ineffective, dysfunctional behavior that is consistently affecting your everyday life has to be dealt with and eliminated.

Start with Yourself

Children, being immature, unformed, and dependent by nature, cannot initiate their own recovery from attention deficit disorder.

The actions and attitudes that ultimately transform the disorder must necessarily start in the adults who care for them. "Change begins within" is a fundamental tenet of the holistic approach to A.D.D.—and since we cannot change the insides of another person, we must necessarily *begin within ourselves*. This idea, while paradoxical, holds true for spouses of A.D.D./A.D.H.D. adults as well.

Lost in Time and Space

Before we begin exploring the process of recovery, we need to understand A.D.D./A.D.H.D. on the levels of mind, body, and energy. If you lend your imagination to the following fantasy, you will get a feeling for what people with A.D.D./A.D.H.D. go through *every day of their lives.*

Imagine that you are the proud owner of a beautiful new car, a car with all the features you've ever wanted in a vehicle. This car is the perfect size, shape, and color for you. When you drive it, you feel safe, in control, and happy, free to go wherever you want or need to go.

Now imagine that you pull into the parking lot of your local mall, park your car, and go inside. You get involved in shopping and forget all about the car. You make some purchases and then happily head back to the car to go home, but in the parking lot, your heart skips a beat: your car is gone.

You stand there, hardly believing your own eyes. You look up and down the row where you thought you parked, but you still don't see your car. Your heart begins to race, and your mind takes off with it. You hope that you are mistaken and are looking in the wrong section of the lot. You begin dashing all over the lot, searching through rows and rows of parked vehicles, desperately seeking your missing car.

During this search, someone you know walks up to you and says hello. She wants to tell you about an upcoming meeting in your town, what it's about, and when and where the meeting will be. You barely hear what she has to say. You can't take anything in because you are too concerned about your lost car.

When she leaves, you realize that you left the keys in the car. Now you feel even worse. Now everything is your fault. Now your mind is spinning negatively, and your body is trembling as the self-recriminating thoughts begin to dominate your thinking.

At one point you spot your car, and a flood of relief runs through you. But when you trot up to it, you see it's not your car. Hoping against hope, you begin retracing your steps, wandering aimlessly around the parking lot, hoping that it's your sense of reality that has been mistaken, but no matter where you look, there's no sign of your car. You feel confused and unhappy, agitated or in a fog. You cannot think clearly and are unable to go anywhere. At heart you blame yourself for your troubles.

A neighbor comes and offers you a ride home in her car. As you ride, she chats about this and that, and you find yourself growing annoyed. You are still thinking about your new car and how you lost it. Though you try to pay attention to what she's saying, you can't. You're feeling so frustrated and upset that your neighbor tries to comfort you, by saying, "You're fine! It's just a car, after all." Though normally polite, you impulsively blurt out a nasty comeback, and that makes you feel even worse. For the rest of the trip, you're filled with feelings of blame and shame. Everything—most of all you yourself—feels so awful and wrong.

A person who is living with ADD/ADHD symptoms experiences the same feelings of frustration, confusion, inadequacy, self-blame, and negativity *every day* of his or her life! Such people are missing something far more valuable than a car, however. They are missing a sense of themselves as positive, competent, or capable people. As a result, they live in a state of more or less on-going turmoil. The out of tune actions and frustrating attitudes are merely reflections of inner confusion about their true identity.

Change will only come when they realize that they possess a powerful inner healing force. When this force is freed and consciously utilized, those who currently suffer from Attention Deficits will begin to create new possibilities for themselves, based on a new self-perspective.

Medical Model Versus Holistic Alternative Approach

Medical

• Symptom is focus of treatment
• Doctor is the sole authority
• Drug is prescribed
• Focus is on the physical
• Goal is symptom removal

Holistic

• Symptom is sign of inner distress
• Clinician is an important ally
• Clinician seeks clues to understand underlying causes
• Patient is active participant in healing process
• Treatment involves life style changes
• Possible use of natural remedies or herbs
• Goal is restoration or transformation to total health

PLEASE NOTE: ADD/ADHD symptoms may also occur from following physical problems: B vitamin deficiency, essential fatty acid deficiency, or iron deficiency, thyroid disorders, exposure to heavy metal pollution, vision issues, autism, Fragile X genetic disorder, and allergens. Please check to rule out these problems when exploring treatment options.

Medical Model Versus Holistic Treatment of ADD/ADHD

Medical

- Goal is to get rid of impulsivity, inattentiveness, and inability to focus, with little input from patient
- Referral to pediatric neurologist
- Occasional referral to psychologist, social worker, mental health counselor
- Little or no follow up

Holistic

- Goal is to transform impulsivity, inattentiveness, and inability to focus by establishing true self-possession of the body, mind and energy levels
- Consultation with school
- Consultation with family
- Family dynamics carefully considered
- Assist parent as role models and leaders
- Encourage child and parents to meet and solve problems using new awareness
- Shift to more wholesome nutrition and lifestyle pattern
- Supplement with tyrosine, B Vitamins, EFA, iron necessary
- Self-sustaining lifelong growth is initiated

ourselves up, supporting and honoring our inner life. This infusion of self-supportive, healing energy in turn empowers us to take on the challenge of overcoming A.D.D./A.D.H.D. in ourselves or in our loved one.

When you are open to healing power, your consciousness is raised, enabling you to see more clearly, communicate more calmly, and take more positive and effective actions. Being open means allowing new ideas to affect us, taking risks by trying out new behaviors until we come to self-sustaining solutions to the problems of A.D.D./A.D.H.D.

Until and unless we are open and start with ourselves, we will not have the power to move the mountain of A.D.D./A.D.H.D., and our loved ones will not have the opportunity to free themselves of the negative patterns and symptoms of the disorder. When we start with ourselves, we come from a place of true authority and self-awareness in our dealings

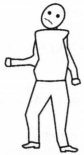

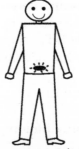

A.D.D./A.D.H.D. Fight or flight response ──▶	Beyond A.D.D./A.D.H.D. Alpha response
Fearful, contracted body	Inwardly calm, expansive
Shallow breathing	Full breathing
"Run" response, speeded up	Self-contained
Hypervigilant	Self-possessed
Muscles rigid, tight	Muscles relaxed
Distant, alienated, alone	Connected, part of process
Frozen, negative, unfocused	Open, positive, focused
Outside	Involved in life experiences
Volatile, reactive	Proactive
Worried	Confident

Moving Beyond A.D.D./A.D.H.D.

From: A.D.D./A.D.H.D. State of Being

All over the place
Living off center
Ungrounded, contracted
Split between mind and body
Seeing the trees but not the forest
Negative mind, negative self-talk
Unable to organize energy to be in the present
Open boundaries, enmeshed, codependent
Need to control
Blaming self and others
Reactive emotions: fear, anger, mood swings
Low self-esteem

To: Self-Containment, Freedom from A.D.D./A.D.H.D.

Self-possessed
Centered
Grounded, expansive
Embodied
Owner of personal space
Body aligned
Positive spirit and resonance
Able to get what is needed
Proactive and efficient
Loving, using negative emotions as signals/fuel
Takes the long view, sees both forest and trees
Selective boundaries
Accepting self and others
High self-esteem

with others. This authority shifts the balance and allows change to occur.

Starting with ourselves means tuning in to ourselves as we move through the day. When we start with ourselves by opening up our healing power, our energy naturally and automatically rises, which in turn enables us to "lighten up." We begin to allow ourselves more pleasure in living as we put the focus on creating a lifestyle that truly reflects us.

A person who is open to new ideas and new energy is capable of being fully present, living in the here and now, bringing all concentration to the moment. His or her actions tend to be appropriate because they are in the right relationship to the self.

In the holistic approach to wellness, inner harmony ultimately creates outer harmony, which in turn leads to genuine connection between people, the bottom line of self-development. By freeing ourselves of old ideas and patterns, we free our loved ones; with our own inner light turned on, we light their way to health as well.

How to Use this Book

If you have been struggling in the dark with A.D.D./A.D.H.D., we want to turn on a light so you can find your way to *your own* healing power, the power that lies in the center of your self. We want to spark your unique creative energies and inspire you to reach inside to your all-knowing, intuitive center so you can reform and transform the negative energy of A.D.D., and replace it with effective living and joy.

Life is too short, and precious childhood time even shorter, for prolonged struggle with the negative symptoms of A.D.D./A.D.H.D.

With the help of the strategies, tools, and techniques in this book, the way will be simple, though not necessarily easy. Take heart, though. The battle you and your loved ones wage against A.D.D./A.D.H.D. will engender strength and power that can be used on every other playing field of life.

We think all readers will benefit from the information in these pages, whether the focus is direct or indirect. Adults with A.D.D./A.D.H.D., for example, are equally advised to read sections addressing the problems (and solutions) parents face, to gain insight about their condition. Likewise, parents will find useful information in the chapter about school (Chapter 10), which speaks directly to teachers. Parents will also find useful information in Chapter 7, "Adults with A.D.D./A.D.H.D.," particularly the discussion of other treatment techniques and modalities. All readers will find a focus on basic themes that when thoroughly understood and put into action will lead them to a life free of A.D.D./A.D.H.D.

Ultimately, your triumph over the disorder will be a gift of lasting value, because in the process of overcoming A.D.D./A.D.H.D. you will have learned, and taught others by your example, to live as a centered, balanced human being, able to perceive, receive, and conceive the best for yourself.

From where we sit, writing this book, across time and space, we are mentally reaching out to you, hoping to join you on the journey to recovery.

Many times, as you follow this path, you will be called upon to face yourself. *This takes courage!* As parents, and as people, we, too, have gone to unproductive, negative places. We still go there at times and have to find our way back, but experience has taught us the skill of getting back home as quickly as possible, bearing the treasure of self-understanding. We wish the same for you.

Right now, it's as if we are all standing on the side of the road, ready for a journey. We, as the authors, can help point out some turns and bumps in the road as we go, but *you are in the driver's seat.*

We want to help you get on the road so you can get moving forward—moving beyond A.D.D./A.D.H.D. We want to be there as you free yourself to live the fulfilling and joyful life you were truly meant to live, enjoying yourself and your family every step of the way.

1

Making Sense of A.D.D./A.D.H.D.

The relationship I have to myself is the relationship I have to my world. It starts with me.

Stanley Keleman, The Human Ground

A.D.D.? That's when nobody's home!

Former patient

The development of a secure, embodied sense of self is the heart and soul of the work to be done to overcome attention deficit disorder, because *as the secure self emerges, the negative symptoms of A.D.D./A.D.H.D. simply fall away, like dead skin.*

The process that creates this miraculous change is the day-to-day work of centering, grounding, sensing one's innermost self, and connecting positively to trusted others. The inner, unseen self is the central force common to all human beings but unique in each. It is the source of all growth, containing all the potential and energy necessary for a rich, full, harmonic, yet individual life experience.

Only when we are centered, grounded, in touch and in tune with this inner self, sensing its needs and supporting it on the inside, can it truly emerge, develop, and, ultimately, flourish.

A full understanding of these key concepts is the underlying theme of this book. But as you explore these ideas, keep in mind that words alone cannot fully communicate truth. Truth—like healing—lies *under* the level of words, in the realm of experience. Our hope and intention is to deliver these ideas in a way that will guide you to the *living experience* of what we're describing.

The old saying that happiness is the journey and not the destination truly applies here; it is the process of discovering the centered core and living securely in the center of one's authentic experience that gives an individual of any age the freedom and the power to move beyond the distressed state of A.D.D. or A.D.H.D.

Good Sense

A close look at the identity of A.D.D./A.D.H.D. people reveals that those who carry the symptoms certainly do not lack potential; on the contrary, they are often creative, talented, full of energy. Most, in fact, are bright. What A.D.D./A.D.H.D. people lack—figuratively, and literally, as we shall later see— is good sense. *They lack a secure sense of themselves as the primary power in their lives.*

Lost in time and space, with mind and body disconnected, they seem unable to accurately or objectively assess their strengths, possibilities, and limitations. Consequently, they fall into the gap between intention and proper action. Unaware of their bodies, and ungrounded on the physical and mental energy levels, they are poor receptors of what is happening in the outside world. In other words, they are out of tune both with themselves and with other people.

A.D.D./A.D.H.D. people go through their days and nights spinning in a negative vortex. Unable to define themselves positively, and lacking awareness of their inner needs, they impulsively act out their feelings or get lost inside themselves. The inner organizer, the part of a person that processes thought into action, is missing, and in its place are anxiety, fear, and negativity.

No wonder the actions of A.D.D./A.D.H.D.-identified people are sometimes self-destructive or irresponsible. This negative behavior occurs because their fundamental relationship to themselves is flawed: *If you have no idea who you are at the core, how can you possibly know what is expected of you, and how to act responsibly? If you have no idea who you are at the core, how can you be anything but ill at ease or anxious?* The A.D.D./A.D.H.D.-identified person is missing the grounding and centering that give comfort and security to the inner self.

The lack of self-possession that creates the misery of A.D.D./A.D.H.D. is a problem of stalled or derailed development on the mind, body, sensing, and energy levels. Exploring each component of this development derailment—as well as what can be done to get the A.D.D./A.D.H.D. person moving forward again—is the focus of this and the next two chapters.

We begin by looking at the process of how people develop a healthy and secure sense of self—one that is centered in the person's own, authentic experience. In the next chapter, we put the focus on *physical and mental grounding* and true *embodiment*, since the way we use our bodies both reflects and creates our inner state. How we connect to others and deal with the discordant aspects, as adults with A.D.D./A.D.H.D. or as the guardians of those who carry the symptoms of the disorder, is explored in Chapter 3. In Chapter 6, we also look at the world of sensory awareness in order to understand how the sensing of the A.D.D./A.D.H.D. person affects his or her ability to accurately perceive, receive, and conceive the world outside.

All of these factors—centering, grounding, connecting, and sensing—are vital to a full understanding of A.D.D./A.D.H.D. *These are the tendrils of A.D.D./A.D.H.D. that must be untangled, one by one, if we are to free ourselves or help others free themselves from the disorder.* Each of these factors affects one's ability to connect and relate to oneself at the most essential level of being. Only when we are grounded, embodied, self-aware, and self-accepting, taking in from our senses and giving out from a secure sense of self, can we be said to be in the right relationship to ourselves.

> *I believe*
> *The greatest gift*
> *I can conceive of having*
> *from anyone*
> *is to be seen by them,*
> *heard by them*
> *to be understood and*
> *touched by them*
> *The greatest gift*
> *I can give is*
> *to see, hear, understand*
> *and to touch*
> *another person*
> *When this is done*
> *I feel contact has been made.*
>
> *Virginia Satir*

Moving beyond A.D.D. means using all your faculties—*mental, physical, and sensory*—in the process of creating change.

Developing in the Right Relationship

In love, when people find the "right relationship," it means they've found someone comfortable to be with, who meets their needs at a very basic level. Having found the right relationship, people become stronger, free to grow and develop and to move forward in life.

The concept of being in the "right relationship" to one-self is very similar. Being in the right relationship to yourself means being at home in yourself, on a body, mind, and energy level. It's a state of being fully conscious, fully present, and comfortable at the core.

To begin thinking about the process of developing this capacity, picture a well-cared-for baby lying in a crib. He does not yet think; he senses. He senses the need to connect outside himself, and to be fed.

When connection and feeding are provided in a positive way, the baby stays in the right relationship to himself. His body and sensing self are intact, his senses are integrated, and the developmental process can move forward.

Moving Beyond A.D.D./A.D.H.D. Wheel

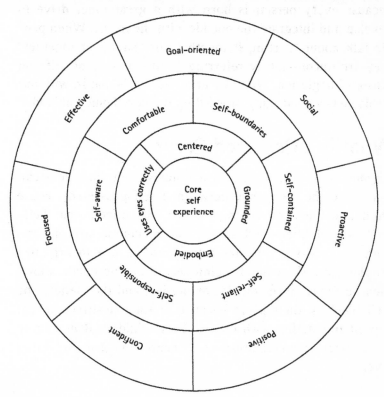

Being in the "Right Relationship" to Oneself

Breathing is complete.
Breathing extends throughout the body.
The body is aligned.
Inner and outer experience are congruent.
A feeling of aliveness prevails.
The person is capable of sensing.
The person is self-possessed.
Consciousness can rise.
The person can fulfill his or her potential.

No one has to teach a baby to crawl, stand, or climb, because every person is born with a great inner drive to develop and integrate the outside with the inside. When people talk about "getting it together" or "having it together" they are unconsciously referring to this process of self and sensory integration. When we are "together"—that is, with our needs met—we naturally proceed up the developmental ladder.

What Is a Centered Core?

Anyone who spends time in a kindergarten classroom can easily see the difference between a self-possessed, secure child and one who is ungrounded and uncentered. Self-possessed children—and adults, too, of course—are at ease. They move easily and are fully present, able to organize around the task at hand. Being secure on the inside allows them to focus on the outside as needed, and they tend to be well liked by their peers because of their positive, upbeat way of interacting with others. These children demonstrate the outward manifestation of a secure and growing inner core.

Whether grown up or still growing, a person with a secure sense of self at core is well balanced. Inner space and outer experience are in harmony and in the right relationship within his or her innermost being.

A calm, centered core, or secure sense of self, is the place where we're at home with ourselves, *regardless of what others think.* It is the place where we are authentically ourselves, being ourselves without embellishment or fear.

Having a secure core means knowing who we are. It means accepting ourselves as imperfect but valuable people, who are in touch with our internal power to grow and change. A secure self is a level of being that goes deeper than the level of personality; it lies *underneath* the personality, at the very center of the self.

In persons suffering from the symptoms of A.D.D., this secure core is felt only by its absence. It is the missing key, the empty hole, and the source of misery. *No amount of stars on the blackboard or doses of medication will ever make up for its absence.*

Creating a Healthy Core: the Eight "C" Factors

In the ideal world—which doesn't exist, of course—all of us would have glowingly healthy cores that developed naturally through the *contact, connection, consistency, comfort, containment, collaboration,* opportunity for *constructive* skill building, and *commitment* that would have been provided to us from the earliest stage of life and onward.

Our parents and caretakers would have been in close loving, and respectful physical *contact* with us from infancy forward. They'd be so secure and unstressed that they'd naturally be tuned in to us, too, providing us with a deep sense of positive, emotional *connection.*

In this perfect world, the adults would make our development easier by providing us with perfectly *consistent* boundaries and guidelines to help us learn and grow, day by day and year by year. Not only that, the whole of society would offer these same safe, consistent boundaries. Adults would also know how to soothe and *comfort* themselves, and therefore would naturally show us how to comfort ourselves when life's stresses appeared.

And of course, any immature, angry, aggressive feelings and outbursts we ever displayed would be calmly *contained* by the strong, secure grown-ups around us—who, by the way, would never be subject to such outbursts themselves.

As we grew, the adults around us would *collaborate* with us, too, bringing us in on the decision-making process in an appropriate way, and respecting our input.

They would also provide us with plenty of opportunity to participate in *constructive skill-building* activities, which would help us gain the mastery that leads to secure self-esteem.

Yes, parents and caretakers would demonstrate nothing but total *commitment* to their children's growth and development, and there would never be any clashes of needs and desires to interfere with that complete commitment.

Ah . . . if only . . .

Well, as we return to the real world, it's easy to see how the eight essential elements necessary for developing a healthy core are interfered with.

Parents are imperfect. They get tired. They become stressed. They have financial concerns. They may have reached the age of adulthood without attaining complete maturity. They have been raised by other imperfect people, and consequently learned imperfect parenting techniques. Mothers and fathers don't always get along, they have different ideas about discipline.

The Eight "C"s

Input	Output
Contact	Self-Regard
Connection	Self-Reflection
Consistency	Self-Regulation
Comfort	Self-Regard
Containment	Self-Regulation
Collaboration	Self-Respect
Constructive Activity	Self-Reliance
Commitment	Self-Responsibility

Even the deep commitment most parents feel toward their children can sometimes compete with their commitment to their jobs, spouses, or other important components of living.

Contact

Contact is being there—being there on a mind, body, and energy level. The physical contact so necessary to an infant's healthy development becomes the hug we give a second-grader, and the pat on the back we give our teen as he goes out the door. It's the respectful way we listen to a nine-year-old's complaints about a friend. It's having meals with our children.

In our busy technological society contact can be lost, often without our even being aware of it. An example is the plastic baby carriers in which we transport our infants. These youngest and tenderest human beings need the warmth and protection that being close to some*body* provides. An infant who spends an excessive amount of time out of contact with that human warmth may become cut off and overwhelmed by the size and scope of the world he or she has entered. Babies need lots of holding, cooing, and response for their development, and so do older children, even those who appear to reject or shy away from physical contact. They need to know we're there.

Connection

Connection is the quality of "being there." True connection is a deep emotional bonding that comes when people know they are accepted and loved despite any flaws or imperfections. In true connection, there is no need for masks or pretense. Eyes meet, and communication is direct and honest.

Connection comes with the deep knowing that one is thought to be trustworthy and good through and through. Supportive words may help build connection, but *the feeling itself is beyond words.*

In the stress and hurry of modern life, it's easy to forget about this most basic need. Parents need to pay the bills and get the food on the table. From their adult perspective, they may assume a sense of connection with a child that is not mutual. This happens when parents lose sight of developing children whose needs are constantly shifting and changing.

To be connected requires that we stop the action of our lives for a moment and fully take in the other person in a nonjudgmental, accepting way.

Consistency

In human development, consistency creates security. Consistency is reliability of rules, regulations, and routines. It provides the developing person with a strong framework to begin the development process and is an important part of the grounding that we will explore in this book.

When the ground rules are constantly shifting and changing, how can young people know what is expected of them? When there are no reliable rituals or routines to anchor a developing life, how will they be able to develop consistency within themselves?

Comfort

Comfort is the product of human kindness. It's the necessary warmth and soothing that allow us to move forward despite the stresses and strain of living. Comfort can be provided only by someone who is connected to us and who has the empathy to see another's need for comfort.

The problem is that we adults sometimes forget the tender state of childhood feelings. What seems a small discomfort to us may be a large hurt to a developing child. We are not suggesting that people who are developing need coddling. Coddling takes power from people and ultimately gives them a sense of unrealistic expectations of others. True comfort, on the other hand, empowers people to face their hurt and fear, and then free themselves of it.

A young girl with a pricked finger who is told, "Stop crying over a tiny cut like that!" will not learn to soothe herself properly and, consequently, will not learn to regulate her feelings. The child who hears a kind, empathic response, such as, "Ouch! That must hurt, but we'll fix it," has a much better chance of being able to comfort herself, and consequently to tolerate the inevitable upsets that will occur in the future.

Containment

Containing strong, unpleasant emotions, such as anger or fear, is necessary for healthy human development. Through the process of containment, a developing person ultimately learns to tolerate strong feelings and to control any destructive or negative impulses that arise from them. This kind of containment leads to the ability to channel strong feelings into constructive words and actions, freeing the person to move forward in life.

One of the secrets of containment, however, is that it can be learned only by example. Arguing, lecturing, rewarding, and punishing do not go far in teaching a young person to contain strong feelings or negative impulses. For true containment, the adult must be able to contain his or her own strong emotions and avoid taking destructive action. When the adults are able to contain their strong feelings, a safe environment is available for the child to learn to appropriately express his or her own negative feelings, too.

In the heat of upsetting moments, containment can easily be lost as the adult gets swallowed up by the negative energy of the child. What is required then is stepping back, creating a loving separation of the child from the behavior, so that discipline or guidance can be effective. Only a centered, grounded adult can deliver messages of containment that will get the desired results, for the child then has a living example of how to contain and conduct himself during times of emotional upheaval.

Collaboration

The need for collaboration with our developing young ones is an often overlooked and yet crucial ingredient of healthy development. The process of collaboration fundamentally shows respect for the child, which in turn leads to self-respect. Children who are consulted and collaborated with become empowered to know themselves and what they need. During a collaboration, the child is asked to come up with positive, creative solutions to life's challenges, a process that will serve him or her throughout life.

For the A.D.D./A.D.H.D.-identified child, this process is especially important because it counteracts low self-esteem. Asking the child or A.D.D.-identified adult questions such as, "What will keep you on target?" or "How can you help yourself to focus?" or "What can you do to help yourself when you get mad?" will yield good results and aid the person in developing a secure inner core.

Constructive Activity

Self-esteem ultimately comes not from praise, but rather from being capable. Capability in turn develops from learning and practicing skills through constructive activities. The development of technological entertainment has had a profound effect on this area of our lives, and especially on our children's lives. In previous generations, people had to "do" in order to learn or even entertain themselves. Often, in our time, little is required of a child beyond being well behaved; nevertheless, the need to develop skills and busily occupy oneself is as vital to the development of a healthy sense of self as it ever was. Busy children are happy children, and this principle applies to A.D.D./A.D.H.D. children very strongly; they need more, not less, stimulation in order to develop properly.

Commitment

When you add up all these factors—contact, connection, consistency, comfort, containment, collaboration, and the need to provide constructive activity—the sum is a sense of firm and secure commitment to the developing human being. Commitment is the rock-solid sense that no matter who, no matter how, no matter what it takes, the caregiver is going to be there, helping the child to find the best inside him- or herself and develop it step by step.

When the adults in a child's life are strongly committed, the child knows it deep in his or her heart. Similarly, a lack of commitment is felt as well. Think about the angry parent who threatens to send a child away if he doesn't "shape up" or "behave." In that moment, the parent is undermining the child's sense of self by showing a profound lack of commitment to the child's development.

Raising children or growing up as adults requires a tremendous amount of commitment, and moving beyond A.D.D./A.D.H.D. takes even more commitment on top of that! So, it's important to keep in mind that the payoff is tremendous, too. The results of your strong commitment will be nothing less than the development of a strong, secure, and healthy sense of self in your A.D.D./A.D.H.D. loved one.

Unmet Needs—Stopping the Process of Emergence

We've seen—and we all sense—how having our needs for the eight "C" factors fulfilled frees us to move forward in life. This forward movement is the natural process of emergence from inner space to outer space. Gradually, in an atmosphere of safety and comfort, the person whose potential was within the seed of an infant can emerge, grow, and even flower. When the basic conditions are met, the mind and body will naturally be aligned and united, allowing self-awareness and self-organization to become fully functional and effective.

But what happens when the basic needs haven't been met? Then the developing person is not in harmony, and not free to grow. The person grows distant from his or her true center, as if frozen and stuck, living on the edge of experience. The body is not in alignment, the mind is uneasy, and the person's internal experience of self is fragmented or unformed.

Unmet needs have a way of taking precedence over all other factors in our consciousness. Imagine for a moment that as you're reading this book you are very hungry. You would not be able to concentrate on your reading for very long. The need to eat would pull you away from the experience.

Now imagine that as you read this book someone interrupts you to say, "Why are you reading that stupid book? What's wrong with you?" You would probably feel belittled. Your need to feel good about yourself would be unmet, and you'd begin to feel uncomfortable. Chances are that your mind would take off, commencing a negative commentary, forcing you away from your intended task—to read.

It's ironic that the same inability to concentrate would hold true if the person had complimented or praised you for reading. If someone said, "Aren't you just wonderful for reading that book!" your attention would *still* be drawn away, and your concentration broken.

While reading, you have a need to be left alone to read. That need, and all other needs—to eat, to feel OK about yourself—must be met before you can pay attention to reading. Unless and until you are tuned in to yourself and comfortable, with no unmet needs at the moment, you will not have the energy to concentrate on reading or any focusing task.

Unmet needs are always there, affecting the quality of our lives, but as they pile up, the system tries to keep them out of conscious awareness. In time, they will either explode as an outburst, or implode as an awful feeling inside. In either case, *they send us very far from the present moment, and into the sphere of self-disorganization.* The burden of unmet needs essentially stops the forward-moving developmental process necessary for positive living.

For many A.D.D./A.D.H.D. children, the explosion or implosion will happen at school, where they are being asked to stand responsibly on their own two feet. Since leaving home and feeling competent and masterful has not been in the picture, they will lack the wherewithal to do so.

The person who grows with unmet needs gets thrown off the developmental track of full emergence. The unmet needs will even have replaced a healthy body sense, creating a situation in which the person is said to be "up in his head" instead of being rooted in his body space, in the present moment.

An extreme example of this is the schizophrenic, who is lost inside him- or herself, disoriented about time, place, or person. The psychotic is living out an intense lack of connection and rootedness to his or her own secure sense of self, unable to be self-aware, or conscious, in the present moment.

It is sad that some individuals cannot be at their highest potential, experiencing the success of being able to take charge of themselves, and feeling good about themselves and their life experiences. The gift of a secure self is our birthright as human beings. No wonder the A.D.D./A.D.H.D. person who is out of touch with his or her inner self, and living at the mercy of poorly understood, unmet needs, often "feels like I'm going nuts."

It is indeed sad, but we must face the difficult truth—this is what it's like to live with the symptoms of A.D.D./A.D.H.D.

Dylan

When Dylan went to high school, his behavior reflected his inner unmet need for connection. He didn't have any self-boundaries and managed to create a stream of chaos wherever he went. Lacking self-structure within, he constantly tested the environment, confronting his teachers and even intimidating them. To compensate for his lack of inner control, he held himself together by controlling others. Even when he liked a teacher, he would give her a hard time, as if by rote!

The more he got negative reactions, the more he acted out, setting up a vicious cycle that was hard to break. Dylan was not truly free because his energy was imprisoned inside, mired in negativity, and his body could not support staying "on task." The very thing he needed—genuine connection—became harder and harder to attain.

Only when a person has a sense of self can he relate freely to the outside world and to others in an expansive, positive way. When he feels insecure or empty inside, his inner discomfort will take over his consciousness. Instead of developing himself—the self he is not in touch with—he will constantly be looking to fill in the gaps.

When filling in the gaps, there's a tendency to project negativity onto the people with whom he interacts. The negativity thus endowed in others is the mental representation of his disconnection and neediness inside. Dylan has become blind to himself and his actions, and this blindness has become habitual and self-perpetuating.

Too Many Moments Like These Derail Development

On the whole, parents of A.D.D./A.D.H.D. children are warm, kindhearted, conscientious, and loving. Their commitment to their children is often inspiring. Nevertheless, because of outside and inside influences that affect every one of us, disturbances can arise, causing needs to go unmet.

The scenarios that follow are based on composites of people who have brought their children in for treatment. Remember that incidents such as these only exacerbate A.D.D. symptoms when they are multiplied over time.

1. Unmet Need: To Experience for Oneself, to Reach

Firstborn, eight-month-old Matthew is playing on the floor in the living room as his devoted young parents, Sarah and Dave, watch. Matthew spies a rattle lying near his dad's legs. Looking anxious, Sarah pipes up, "He wants the rattle, Dave—give it to him!"

Dave quickly pushes the rattle into Matt's hand. "Sorry, little buddy. Here you go."
Matt looks confused but takes the rattle.

In this scenario, two loving but oversolicitous parents have inadvertently interrupted their son's development by interfering with his doing for himself. Matt, in wanting the rattle, needed to find out how to get it. For instance, he needed to find out that waving his arms around wouldn't get him what he wanted, and that he'd have to stretch and reach to attain his goal.

By getting the rattle for him, his parents unwittingly robbed Matt of an experience of self-accomplishment, the kind that promotes a healthy sense of self and physical embodiment.

In truth, Sarah's internal reaction about having been too often frustrated as a child has clouded her ability to sense Matt's true need. David, too, is anxious to please and show what a good dad he intends to be.

By the time Matt gets the rattle, he has sensed disharmony between his parents because of it. On top of that, he is no longer sure of who wants him to have the rattle in the first place, since his parents were so intent on his having it. Instead of having an enhanced self-identity, such as, "I am the one who reaches and gets," this moment leaves Matt now looking for structure outside of himself. The convoluted lesson he might learn is: "Mom and Dad want me to hold this rattle."

2. Unmet Need: A Moment of Comfort

Three-year-old Ricky walks into the kitchen for breakfast. His mother, Pamela, is pregnant with her second child. She's preoccupied with her own thoughts (including her ideal vision of what a good mother is) and feelings (need to be prompt for doctor's appointment, pressure to get dressed). Ricky lightly bumps his leg against the chair and reacts with a little cry and an unhappy face.

Because Pamela is feeling pressured and anxious, she puts the cereal in front of him without making eye contact, missing the distress on his face. She turns away quickly to sponge the counter. "Hurry up! Eat what Mommy made you, honey!"

A Ricky who is moving toward A.D.D. might now withdraw into dawdling.

A Ricky who is moving toward A.D.H.D. might tip the cereal over "on purpose."

In this scenario, we see clashing needs. Ricky needs a calm, centered mom. Pam needs to organize herself and get out the door.

Pamela is seeing her child through *her mind's eye.* She is not truly seeing him in present-moment consciousness. Her ideal notion of motherhood includes cooking hot cereal and keeping a clean house; her ideal notion of herself is to be prompt for all appointments.

In other words, Pamela is *thinking* herself—that is, she is up inside her head, caught up in her internal pressures, a state in which she is essentially cut off from her own needs and from her child.

If she were *sensing* herself, her inner awareness would lead her to slow down so that she could tune in to Ricky's need for comfort and companionship as well as handle her need to get ready to leave, giving both their due. Pamela needs to learn that the knot inside her stomach is a signal to slow down, calm herself, and get centered.

3. Unmet Need: To Share Oneself

Six-year-old Nicky brings crayons to the table and begins to draw. His mother, Julie, who is putting away groceries, reacts as if shining a bright spotlight on him. "Oh, wow, look at you! You're draw-

ing!" He holds up a picture. "Isn't that great! Oh, you're so great. Just great!"

When her husband, Joe, walks in, she continues. "Look what Nicky drew! Isn't it great?"

With barely a glance, Joe remarks enthusiastically, "That's really great, Nick!"

Instead of feeling strengthened and confident, Nicky now feels unsettled. He didn't think the picture was great; he was just showing it to share a part of himself with his mother. Now he has doubts. Maybe it *is* great and he can't tell. Maybe it's *not* great and he fooled his mother (which makes him feel as if he did something wrong). Maybe if he does another drawing, they won't like it. If he does art again, he may do it to get attention and not from a spontaneous impulse. Feeling uncomfortable, Nicky hops from the table and runs away.

Julie has hardly seen her son's artwork because what is dominant in her thinking is her need to be a good mother by praising Nicky. When she and Joe were children, they were not praised very much. Now they want to make up for lost time, with Nick. In the process, because they are focusing on their internal images of being good parents, but not on *sensing* themselves and their own needs they have lost perspective. Unwittingly, Julie and Joe have lost touch with the real moment and their real son.

4. Unmet Need: Discipline and Containment of Negative Impulses

Ten-year-old Peter is in a "bad mood" because he had a conflict with another student in school. That night, at home, Peter makes an unprovoked attack on his younger brother Nathan, who was given a special school award for a story he composed. Peter steals Nathan's notebook, rips out the pages, and stuffs them in the toilet, laughing. When he is discovered, he makes up a story about Nathan having stolen his special pencil first.

When Nathan complains, Andrea, the boys' mom, tells Peter not to touch his brother's notebook again. She gives Peter a time-out, sending him to his room for five minutes. Nathan is frustrated and furious but feels powerless; he knows his mother never really punishes Peter.

Later that night, Andrea has a long discussion with Peter in his bedroom, analyzing his feelings about the incident at school and about his brother winning the contest. She effectively helps Peter to rationalize and make excuses for his bad behavior.

In this scenario, Andrea is very invested in Peter's being right, because she fears that her son's bad behavior makes her a bad mother. Because of this, she can never allow herself to see him as less than her idealized image of him. As a consequence, she diminishes her true feelings and covers up what is real, never fully experiencing the negative side of Peter's acting out. Because she is unconscious of Peter's negative behavior, she doesn't act in a powerful, appropriate way when Peter needs to be put in his place.

When she is disciplining, her eyes, voice, and body position are so weak that the unspoken message is that bad behavior will be tolerated. Another hidden factor here is that as a child Andrea was highly controlled and consequently became a goody-goody who never misbehaved. Therefore, deep inside since the time Peter was a toddler, she has derived a certain amount of pleasure from his mischievousness and has unwittingly rewarded him for it by giving him attention or by letting him believe his misdeeds were cute when he was younger.

Carl, Peter's father, would like to be firmer, but he knows from experience that disciplining Peter upsets Andrea very much. In addition, Carl's father used to come down so hard on him that Carl automatically went to the other extreme, avoiding giving discipline. So, Carl too steps back—when he's around, that is—which is less and less often, given the emotional climate at home.

How Peter longs for his place and his own self-structure. But the more he looks for it, by controlling the family with his bad behavior, the more it eludes him. Peter is even aware that he has more power than his father. That makes him feel scared and guilty. And so, he provokes more and more each day, on an uncontrolled, self-perpetuating path that brings his self-esteem down. His simple, all-driving need to know his place is constantly thwarted.

To the extent that this pattern has continued throughout Peter's childhood, he and his family are in trouble. As a child, Peter cannot understand his behavior, let alone change it. His parents will have to take the lead by looking at their own part in the family dynamics. Peter can change his negative behavior only when Andrea and Carl change their responses to it. This means looking under the surface of the family dynamics and unraveling the facade of normalcy that disguises their unhappiness with each other.

If this seems too daunting a task, they may need to give themselves permission to seek professional help in clarifying the patterns and dynamics that reinforce or allow Peter's naughty behavior.

5. Unmet Need: To Discover for Oneself

Stuart and Anna have taken seven-year-old Brad on a day's outing to a local amusement park. Instead of focusing on having a good time, they are focusing on Brad's having a good time.

They constantly point things out to him. "Look, Brad, there's the Ferris wheel!" "Look at that ride, Brad!" "Hey, Brad, look at the arcade!" "Look, Brad, there's the merry-go-round!"

Poor Brad. He hasn't had a chance to discover anything for himself. Without understanding why, he feels cranky and begins acting petulant and demanding on the ride home.

"I don't know what's wrong with that kid," his father later complains. "We do everything for him, but he's never happy."

This pattern has been on going since Brad was a tot. In their desire to fulfill their notions of good parenting, his parents inadvertently took over Brad's space and experience, stealing his ability to discover who he is on his own. As Brad's frustration has risen, so has his negative acting out behavior.

Adult loves "too much" → interrupts experience → disrupts person's emergence → low self-esteem

Sensing Oneself	Vs.	Split Off from Oneself
Embodied		Up in the head
Tuned in to inner needs		Unaware of inner needs
Fully present in the moment		Listening to internal chatter
In touch with inner self		Out of touch with inner self
Open to new ideas		Rigid about new ideas
Body is comfortable		Body is out of awareness
Thinking is clear		Thinking is defensive
Truly knows and senses self		Thinks about self

My Inner Unmet Need + Your Inner Unmet Need =
A Negative Interaction Between Us

Go deep inside yourself
Find that treasure that
Is known by your name.

Virginia Satir

Relationship of Thought and Action

Effective Functioning: Thought—(Pause)—Action

- Action follows thought (ideals or goals) naturally and automatically
- Gets job done effectively with least "pause" or time delay
- Optimal movement; gets results; usually successful at getting what is needed or wanted
- Breathing is full and deep
- Embodied and connected: muscles are relaxed

A.D.D. Functioning:
Thought . . . (Pause) . . . Action

- Too long a delay between thought and action
- Daydreaming, distant
- Disembodied, tuned out
- Little movement, stuck
- Shallow breathing
- Muscles untoned

A.D.H.D. Functioning:
Thought—Action (No pause, no reflection)

- No pause between thought and action
- Reaction substitutes for intention in effort to reduce anxiety
- Movement is chaotic, scattered, all over the place
- Too much action, can't stay in one place
- Muscles are rigid, tight

Hope into Power

There is so much hope, if we start with ourselves! When we become conscious and have the courage to carefully look at ourselves as the source of our experience, not in a blaming or self-deprecating manner but rather as a way of cleaning house, then hope will rise and transform into power.

With the windows wide open, fresh air can breeze in. We have seen almost miraculous change when people stop looking outside themselves to other people, or to foreign substances, and reclaim their power by connecting to their bodies and seeking their answers within.

According to the holistic tradition, the outer conditions of life ultimately reflect the inner conditions of the heart. When we can drop our ego investment in being right, blaming, or knowing it all, we can begin a search for real truth. Because our focus is in the right place, everything will proceed, and we'll find our truths along the way.

According to the wisdom of the Hawaiian huna healing system, where attention goes, energy flows. This elusive but obvious truth is very hopeful when attention is given to gaining the knowledge, patience, and wisdom needed to help yourself or a loved one move beyond A.D.D. You can be sure that positive energy will begin and flow inside you, strengthening you for upcoming challenges. When gaining wisdom and overcoming negativity become the focus, how freeing the truth will be!

2

Going Within—
the New Frontier

*No shrine is holier than the human frame, for it houses
the human spirit.*

Majid Ali, M.D.

Picture lightning, crackling through the night sky, a zigzag
flash, and a crash of thunder. Lightning is electrical energy
that is fierce, wild, and uncontrolled. If it strikes someone,
that person could be destroyed by its sizzling power. If it
strikes a building, it can cause it to burst into flames.

Now imagine a beautiful city lit up at night by the same
power of electricity. Because the citizens of the city have
light, they are able to work and play. Here, electrical energy
has been *focused*. It's a useful and positive power. Walking
under a brightly glowing street lamp, we would feel safe from
harm. The electricity would guide us and light our way.

The difference between these two phenomena is *energy
organization*. Electricity needs to be organized or *grounded*
in order to be useful, effective, and positive. And so do
human beings.

To be grounded as a human being means to be comfortable with one's innermost self, and to have boundaries. It
means knowing where we start and where we end; accepting ourselves as imperfect but valuable individuals. It means
being contained, embodied, and tuned in to our innermost

self on a deep, instinctual level. Being grounded also allows us to live in the center of our own experience, expanding our energy outward from a secure base.

Every human being is an energy system, both literally and figuratively. This human energy system moves constantly in time and space, forming and organizing itself, expanding and contracting. It follows that when the energy system is connected and organized, the person inside can emerge, expand, and grow consistently, connecting to others in an appropriate, positive way.

But when the system is inwardly focused on unmet needs or perceived inadequacies, the result is imbalance, a spinning out of control in search of self-structure "out there," or an inward retreat from others.

An adult or child afflicted with attention deficit disorder is like an ungrounded electrical circuit. The person's energy system may send out sparks of hyperactivity, or simply short-circuit on the inside, causing a breakdown through lack of focus and attention. Either way, such people are unable to organize their internal space and connect with themselves or others on a healthy, fully functioning level.

Grounding our precious human energy so that it works to light our way is what moving beyond A.D.D./A.D.H.D. is all about.

The way a person uses his or her body is an often ignored but powerful determinant of the person's inner and outer experience. Since the mind and body operate like mirrors, reflecting the same truth, a lack of focus in a person's mental life shows up in the physical structure.

Moving beyond A.D.D. involves a shift in the way a person uses his or her body and senses. It starts with the development of an organized, centered, and grounded *self.*

Missing in Action

As a result of their difficulty sensing themselves in their body space, A.D.D./A.D.H.D. people are disempowered and consequently are on shaky ground in life. What's lacking is a basic comfort and confidence level within. They literally do not feel at home in their minds or their bodies. Instead they are lost in a maze of inner unfulfilled needs that keep them disembodied, dependent, and fragmented. Whether this manifests as the fog of A.D.D. or as the frenzy of hyperactivity, the essential self of an A.D.D. sufferer is truly missing in action.

> *To have form*
> *is to be alive*
> *But to remain fixed*
> *in a form*
> *is to stagnate*
> *Our destiny is to*
> *continue to form.*
> *Stanley Keleman*

What's really missing, however, is a developmental process. Instead of growing a stable, secure sense of self, the A.D.D./A.D.H.D. person is left holding the pieces of his or her fragmented, underdeveloped self. No wonder the assumption of personal control is so difficult and foreign in such a case.

It is possible to get the process of development back on track, as people learn to center and ground themselves and to begin to integrate the previously discussed "C" factors. Nevertheless, we first need to understand and demystify the negative behavioral aspects of A.D.D./A.D.H.D. in order to achieve greater compassion for the person caught in its trap.

Though people in the grip of the disorder may valiantly "try" to control themselves, their efforts are doomed because *there is no firmly rooted self to control.* Their predicament is mirrored in the body and can include any number of sensory problems, such as avoidance of eye contact, eye focus difficulties, auditory confusion, and tactile disturbances.

On the physical level we predictably will see disharmony between head and body, with head flopping over as the person sits at a desk trying to concentrate, or head held rigid with tight neck muscles. The sense of intentionality is lost, too, as arms and legs splay out aimlessly, or are pulled in and contracted in an inappropriate self-protective posture.

Bridging the Gap

Shifting self-perception and physical alignment is like standing at the water's edge contemplating plunging in. As you face the water, your thinking mind begins to race, filling in the gap between your intention of swimming and the action of swimming. If you are stuck, your thoughts tend to be negative. You think, *the water's too cold; what if I don't like it?*

At some point either you will fall back, away from your intention, by going back to your blanket, or the tension will build up, propelling you forward to take the plunge.

The gap between thinking and doing is the energy place of self. If you, as an embodied person, bridge the gap of action and intention by plunging in, you will truly experience yourself in the moment. You will become the experience of swimming, sensing your body, and correctly perceiving yourself, the water, and the experience of swimming.

The problem is that the A.D.D./A.D.H.D. person falls into the gap between intention and action because she is not truly embodied. Consequently, she remains distant, stuck and frozen, at the edge of experience. She unconsciously removes herself mentally by drifting up into her head like an unanchored boat, or flees her discomfort, in a futile attempt to run away from the feelings of emptiness inside.

Billy

Billy was four and a half years old and "wired." His muscles were like tight rubber bands and he could not stay in one place for a minute. He had been put out of three nursery schools because the teachers didn't know where to begin with him. He had no center, anchor, or inner space from which to process himself.

Very quickly I (Rita) started to establish his connection to his body by having him take a deep breath and sense his feet firmly on the ground. I asked him to look outside at a particular tree and explained that, in a way, people are like trees—they need to be rooted. Like trees they need to reach up, too, all the way to the stars. After Billy stood and reached, his feet secure to the ground, his body started to relax and soften, and he started to breathe more fully, literally slowing himself down, and connecting to himself. "Now you are calm. Now *you* can choose what you want to do first," I said.

As he slowed down, he became a different person. He began to stay with his experiences in playing, which in turn allowed his creativity and exuberance to begin to emerge in an appropriate, natural way.

Considering that he had been bouncing off the walls, a miracle had occurred by the third session: he had learned to press his feet down on the ground, take a breath, and stretch up to calm himself. This experience of self-control was powerful for him. He learned that he could command his impulses and began to open up to his natural state of being.

Later, he noticed a tape player in the corner and asked if we could play some music. He wanted to put the tape in by himself, so I showed him how and let him do it. If I had put the tape in I would have spoiled his experience of doing and robbed him of a chance to experience himself as capable. "You can do it," I told him. "You can trust yourself."

When the music came on, his face lit up. He looked up at me, and our eyes met. We were truly experiencing each other in that moment. He reached up and took my hands, and we began to dance.

A.D.D. and Body Structure

When a person grows and develops naturally, the body also develops, as a living structure that can support the person's ability to experience life fully. Think of someone you know who is self-possessed and confident: the body is aligned, the head and the body move in a harmonious, connected way.

In such a person, the eyes are clear and sparkling, easily meeting the eyes of others, and having full binocular vision. The shoulders are held squarely but not rigid. The upper body is held up, in a relaxed way that allows for deeper breathing. The limbs move in concert with the rest of the body, giving a feeling of grace and harmony. The breath reaches from the Hara point, just below the navel (see Chapter 4), to complete the self-circuit. The lower half of the body is grounded and stable, with legs and feet connected to the floor and the earth, providing a true base for movement and expansion.

A body like the one described naturally reflects a lightness and vibrancy; it exudes an energy that is generally positive, connected, regulated, and strong. Think about the implications of going through life with such a body and mental structure. People who are so well aligned can easily move toward what they want and need; they can withstand frustration and stress. They are not unduly sensitive or focused on what others think is right for them.

Perhaps most important, they can take in information and give out expression in an assertive, confident, secure manner. The body has literally grown over time to become a home for the self, a structure that is supportive and attuned to the person's authentic experience.

How different is the body structure of most A.D.D. and A.D.H.D.-diagnosed people, whose bodies tend to be unattuned and unsupported. In both A.D.D. and A.D.H.D. the body is contracted, shoulders are not squared off, chest is caved in, with shallow breathing, which in turn diminishes the amount of oxygen coming into the brain.

In the case of A.D.D. without hyperactivity, the body appears undercharged. The breath is shallow and the chest caved in. The head and the body move in a disconnected way. The lower half of the body is not grounded to the floor, and often the limbs hang loose, as if disconnected to the rest of the body. The person appears not to have a home in his or her body.

In A.D.H.D. people, we see the same lack of grounding and alignment, but with taut, rigid muscles in an over-charged, overextended, speeded-up system. Such individuals are not self-contained; on the contrary, they need to be in constant motion, compensating for the lack of being at home with themselves.

A.D.D./A.D.H.D. from a Psychostructural Dynamic Perspective

From the psychostructural dynamic (PSD) perspective, A.D.D./A.D.H.D.-identified people are:

- Either codependent, enmeshed, living in the shadow of another; overly dependent, waiting for others to do for them; or falsely independent, acting as if they need no one but feeling inadequate

- Self-alienated, disconnected from their authentic (core) experience

- Frozen inside, rigid and controlling

- Uptight, muscularly tense

- Unaware of personal boundaries, likely to invade others' space

- Constantly testing the environment, in search of structure from the outside

- Impulsive and impatient

- Lacking points of self-reference in the body

- Not tuned in to their self-experience

- Cut off from pleasure, negative, whiney, complaining

- Undefined and disorganized

- Speeded up in an effort to flee internal discomfort

- Living with a distorted relationship to time, living in the past or future

- Blameful of others in a futile attempt to compensate for missing self-structure

- Unrelated to real time, procrastinators, taking too much or too little time

- Missing important root points of body awareness

- Unable to perceive accurately—eyes do not serve seeing, ears do not serve hearing

- Holding the head rigidly or tending to flop over

- Not at home in their body, "nervous" or tuned out, daydreaming

Body, Space, Body Language

A.D.D.-diagnosed children tend to show their symptoms in the way they carry themselves and fill their *body space*. People carrying the symptoms of attention deficit disorder are not *anchored* in their own body, and consequently, they can appear uncomfortable and awkward. They do not experience themselves or get a clear self "feedback." They are split and distant both from their self-organizing body space and from the expansive energy necessary to maintain consistent and persistent movement toward an outside goal.

Helping A.D.D./A.D.H.D. children and adults to become more aware of themselves as unique individuals and true *owners* of their bodies, and the space their bodies occupy, is a vital step toward moving beyond A.D.D. In the initial session at the Center, we state, "[Name], growing up is knowing how to take care of *yourself.*" This galvanizes awareness, attention, and energy on the person's self space.

Though the physical-alignment aspect of A.D.D./A.D.H.D. is often ignored or downplayed, it is key to recovery. A shift in the child's use of his or her body tends to automatically set other positive changes in motion. A person who gains awareness of his or her groundedness will naturally begin to feel more secure in living. The head and body will be in right relationship so that energy is available to see, perceive, and interact with the environment. Attention that has been utilized for holding oneself together is now freed up and available for positive exploration of the world around one.

For example, children who learn to "carry" themselves well gain both self-respect and respect from others. This natural respect for a person who is properly aligned and self-possessed is not something of which most people are consciously aware, but it colors their experience nevertheless. When a self-assured, self-confident person walks down the street, others may unconsciously turn their heads to get a better look. Self-possession in a human being is attractive, and unfortunately, for the A.D.D./A.D.H.D. person, who lacks this important quality, the opposite is true as well.

Nan

If you were to meet Nan now, you would never identify the alert seven-year-old as a formerly A.D.D.-diagnosed child. Highly fearful of attending school, Nan had at first been labeled as "shy" in class, but, despite the teacher's best efforts to make her comfortable, her inability to participate in class failed to change. Her constant daydreaming and inability to make friends soon led to her being an object of ridicule with the other children. The school authorities suggested that Nan be given Ritalin in order to control or mask her negative symptoms. Nan's teacher was con-

cerned that without medication, the child's situation would degenerate from bad to worse.

Nan's mother, Sandy, however, was concerned about the potential long-term side effects of giving her young daughter strong psychopharmaceutical medication, and after receiving a diagnosis of A.D.D. from her medical doctor, she opted for treatment that was medication free.

Nan's problems were clearly visible in the way she occupied, or failed to occupy, her body space. She walked awkwardly and tentatively, held herself tightly, and hardly appeared to breathe. Her shoulders seemed locked and frozen, her chest was caved in, and she held her head down, like a little turtle in a shell. Her eyes were constantly downcast on the floor, totally avoiding contact.

Given her defended and self-conscious use of body space, Nan was not even free to look up, let alone pay attention in class, or participate with other children. She was very sensitive to what the teacher thought and did, and she had no friends. Clearly, her core development was stalled.

Like all A.D.D.-diagnosed children, Nan had also picked up the unspoken message (from the adults in her life) that "there is something wrong with her." *The feeling of defect in the innermost core is the basis of all mental discomfort, and a major factor with A.D.D.-identified people.*

Being dependent and unformed, as all children are, Nan could not possibly know that she lacked a secure sense of self. The work with her began with an eye-opening, clear communication of an opposite point of view:

"Nan, there is nothing *wrong* with you."

This message needs to be communicated loud and clear to all adults and children who exhibit the symptoms of attention deficit disorder. Their behavior might be wrong, they may perceive themselves and others inaccurately, but on the deepest, truest, and most important level of being, there is nothing *wrong* with any of us.

Rita continued, "You are wonderful, and all that you are and can be is within you right now. I'm going to help you get yourself out of the way so that you can see what is working and what's not working in your life. This is like an adventure trip for you to get to know yourself and believe in yourself. It's not about your parents, your teacher, or me. The power lies *in you* to reshape yourself, inside and out, so that you can be all and have all you need to live your life successfully."

Even a young child will understand the meaning of this freeing and empowering message.

In consultation, Nan's mother began to see that she had unwittingly fallen into the trap of overparenting based on her own leftover fears from childhood. Sandy hovered over her daughter in an attempt to avoid the distant, underparenting style of her own mother. She noticed and commented on her daughter's every movement, for instance. Her own self-fear kept her riveted on all Nan's experiences. This fear resonated to Nan in all levels of her being.

As Sandy learned to step back from Nan, literally as well as figuratively, Nan could start to experience herself in a more natural way. She began to take more responsibility for herself and her conduct. Her shoulders seemed to widen, and her step became surer. The natural and harmonious relationship between body and mind that is every human's birthright came into a place of restoration. Nan was learning to literally "stand on her own two feet."

Instead of cowering, Nan's body language now seemed to say, "I'm here. I'm present." Her eyes met the eyes of others freely and without shame. The other children at school perceived the change and began respecting her, which led to other positive changes.

Nan gained the ability to tune in to herself and anchor herself by using the tools and techniques contained within this book.

Connecting Heads to Bodies— the Elusive Obvious

Just as an electrical wire needs to be connected for a machine to run efficiently, so Nan needed to reconnect to her natural state of being. She learned that *breathing deeply and fully would put her in touch with her inner sensing space, the bedrock of self-awareness and consciousness. This is the arena for healing, the elusive obvious ground of being.*

Tuning in to herself on a fundamental level increased both her alertness and calm. Deep breathing sends refreshing oxygen to the brain, increasing concentration and focus. People who are rigid, contracted, or frozen in the way they hold their bodies are not in a position to breathe fully.

As a person takes in more oxygen, gaining awareness of the body as him- or herself, the body circuit naturally reconnects. In the process, the person feels calmer and more in control of thinking and feeling.

People in this state are now able to structure themselves from within and expand into the world because their energy is grounded and organized.

Once in the right relationship to the inner self and to outside experience, the person is capable of being effective, conscious, present, and successful.

3

The Nitty-Gritty

You don't have to know anything to be negative. You have to know a great deal to be positive.

R. Buckminster Fuller

When everyday life is lived under the spell of A.D.D./A.D.H.D., discord and upsets fill far too many of life's precious moments. No life is free of upsetting experiences, of course, but when A.D.D./A.D.H.D. people are involved there are apt to be an intolerable number of power struggles and disappointments.

Only when the discordant aspects of the disorder are thoroughly understood by the A.D.D./A.D.H.D. adult or by parents and teachers of the A.D.D./A.D.H.D. child can change be effected, for understanding in this case means being able to free oneself from the negative dynamics. The goal of this chapter is to promote understanding by illustrating the patterns that underlie the disorder and create the anguish of A.D.D./A.D.H.D.

Parents who come for treatment have often reached a point of no return when it comes to disciplining or motivating their A.D.D./A.D.H.D. children. There is a feeling that nothing works. We hear statements such as:

"He's got me over a barrel."

"I do what the books say to do. But it doesn't work with my A.D.D. child."

"Every day I tell myself I'm not going to lose control, but he knows how to push my buttons, and I wind up losing it anyway!"

Fortunately, this level of frustration need not last a lifetime. When the discordant dynamics that support A.D.D./A.D.H.D. are understood on a mind, body, and energy level, a shift will automatically and naturally occur. The unproductive pattern can then be noticed and eliminated by the most mature party in the relationship. In effect, one party removes him- or herself from the conflict. In A.D.D./A.D.H.D. as in other arenas of human life, "it takes two to tangle," and the removal of one party topples the pattern of conflict.

Think for a moment of two mothers who are putting their eight-year-old children to bed. The first mother—mother A—liked to stay up late as a child but was never allowed to do so. Deep inside, perhaps away from her conscious awareness, she identifies with her child's wish to remain part of the action at night. She directs her child in a halfhearted manner to go to bed, her voice and body stance weak. When he appears in the living room moments later, she allows him to linger, perhaps even rewarding him with the unspoken message that he is cute or appealing.

Because mother A identifies with her child's fear of being alone in his bedroom, she lingers there, too, talking with him, perhaps even reasoning with him about the need to go to sleep. Secretly, there is an aspect of pleasure about spending this time with her child, since she was separated from him all day.

In other words, when setting the limit of bedtime, mother A is pulled off center; she's not really congruent and grounded in her intention to put her son to bed. Unfortunately, this conflict may escalate, resulting in harsh words or unpleasant feelings as her frustration about his wakefulness rises later in the evening.

The second mother, mother B, is centered and grounded about her child's need to get to bed. All parts of her agree that he needs his rest and she needs her evening as an adult. She delivers the message that bedtime is near with inner conviction; her voice and body stance communicate certainty.

If mother B wants to enjoy some time with her child at night she makes sure that the bedtime ritual allows plenty of connection time for both of them. *As she lovingly tucks him in and dims the light, she is tending to her personal needs as well as his.* Mother B realizes that she has both the need and the right to have part of her evening as adult time, just as she is certain that her son needs a good night's rest to function well the next day. There's just no "give" in her position.

If her child were to appear in the living room, he would calmly, lovingly, and firmly be guided back to his bedroom. Because of her congruent, inner conviction—consistently delivered over the years—her child would know the ground rules of bedtime and comply.

For adults with A.D.D./A.D.H.D. the process of moving away from the discordant aspects of the disorder entails commiting the care of the self to the most responsible aspect of oneself, leading with one's sense of even fledgling maturity. The part of the self that is seeking recovery from the disorder can be relied upon to set ground rules and, like a parent, has to become the strong, calm motivator inside.

In the case of children with A.D.D./A.D.H.D., the shift in the discordant pattern has to come first inside the parent or caregiver, who then creates new and healthier interactions that break the old, debilitating behaviors.

How Do You Discipline an A.D.D./A.D.H.D Child?

Let's get this out of the way immediately: Disciplining an A.D.D./A.D.H.D. child has little to do with being strict or being lenient. *A parent who is centered in his or her own expe-*

rience will naturally and automatically deliver discipline in a way that is clear, concise, and effective. Limit-setting and other aspects of discipline and child guidance automatically strengthen on both verbal and nonverbal levels when the parent is standing firm within his or her personal, psychic space.

It happens like this: *When the parent is centered, the child receives the disciplinary message with all the clarity and intention that is behind it and usually complies.* The child drops resistance and resentment because on a deep intuitive level, he or she feels guided or taken care of--not "bossed around" or controlled.

This process works for both parties: because the parent is firmly and securely in the parent place, the child can be put in the child place--and feel secure there, too!

Moreover, with the clarity of centered, grounded disciplining, neither party will have to react to unmet needs. Instead, both parent and child will move toward self-containment and reasonableness. Think for a moment. Who has higher self-esteem, the reasonable person or the unreasonable person?

When parents begin looking after themselves on the most fundamental level and building their lives around what gives them joy, in time--and more quickly than you may think--the child will respond. Children will automatically begin to understand *for themselves* that rules are there not to punish but rather to organize their experience and provide necessary structure.

This idea can be communicated directly to a child by a parent, teacher, or primary care physician through a simple metaphor. "Discipline is like the tires of a car. Without them, the car can never go anywhere, no matter how powerful the engine."

In time, children start to sense that they are individuals, in charge of their own lives, and that discipline is strengthening. When they begin truly living in their own space, no longer in a state of codependency or isolation, their sense of self-responsibility enters the picture.

In other words, the child too will have learned to start with oneself first.

A Walk in the Park

As I (Rita) was walking through Golden Gate Park while visiting my son, I saw examples of how our good intentions as parents can be undermined by our own shadows and incompleteness as people.

I came across a pond with ducks swimming in it and decided to sit down next to an older woman who was semi-dozing in the sun. A small child was standing nearby. The child was experiencing the ducks, the pond, and the water, but she seemed lonely. She smiled at me and I smiled back.

The older woman was her grandmother, who appeared tired and tuned out. Only when the child walked over to play in some nearby bushes did the grandmother come to life. Then she fearfully called to the child to come back. She connected to her grandchild only from a state of fear.

Another family walked by—a mother and father and two young children. The children seemed very happy to be at the water's edge, experiencing the ducks and the pond, but the mother abruptly interrupted the experience, saying, "It's cloudy. Let's come back when it's sunny." The children seemed disappointed as the family turned and left. The mother appeared to miss the fact that there was still much to enjoy even though the day was slightly overcast.

Another mother came by with a child in a stroller. The child looked happy to be in the park, but the mother looked anxious and worried. While gazing at the ducks, the child coughed, and the mother responded harshly, "Learn to cover your mouth when you cough!" The child's face lost its happiness immediately, and the child, too, now seemed anxious.

The point is that we are all imperfect and with good intentions. But many times our leftover, unfulfilled parts overshadow what could be our best experiences. When this happens our loved ones, too, wind up caught in these shadows.

Again, guilt and blame have no role here. No parents can ever be perfect. (Truly perfect parents might be the most horrible burden of all!) What we have to understand is that, *unless we maintain a high degree of self-awareness, we will naturally and automatically act and react according to how we were formed from our earliest childhood experiences. This excess baggage mars present-moment living and interferes with the free, unencumbered, and even joyful connection between people.* It is the work of each of us to see and understand the shadow that we cast over ourselves and our children. Once our inner eyes are open, we can gradually free ourselves of the leftover negative patterns that we are unwittingly passing along to the next generation.

Over- and Underparenting

Parenting is a balancing act. Even with the best intentions, it's a rare parent who hasn't tipped the scales to over- or underparenting. (We certainly have!) No blame or fault is connected to these patterns, but we must be aware of them if we intend to create the safe, nurturing environment that supports the emergence of the child's core self.

Overparenting, a form of codependency, like workaholism, is often esteemed in our society, so it is natural for parents to confuse it with true devotion. Overparenting takes on infinite manifestations, but the tendency is for the parent to invade the child's developing core—to fuss, direct, manipulate, correct, urge, and prompt the child about every little thing. These are the moms and dads who fret about whether a sweater is on or off, and tell the child to whom to say hello and when.

Instead of guiding or leading, they hover. They often do too much for a child—such as dressing, catering to, or bathing a seven-year-old. Some overparenters, perhaps because they believe that a happy child is a sign of good parenting, allow the child's every passing mood to color their own emotional state.

An overparenter may also confuse dependence and clinging with love and actively promote the child's being dependent in a way that's inappropriate for the child's age. (These same patterns apply to spouses of A.D.D./A.D.H.D. adults, who often have parental aspects in their relationships with their mates.)

Underparenting is the other side of the coin, the one that is showing when parents are too stressed out or exhausted to involve themselves with the nitty-gritty details of parenting. The pattern of underparenting, which is more thoroughly discussed later, creates an internal sense of isolation in the child, or loneliness in the adult carrying the symptoms of the disorder.

Other kinds of parenting patterns also produce problems and obstruct the emergence of the child's core self. Consider the following:

- *If a parent is habitually negative,* the child's core will not develop properly in an attempt to defend itself from parental criticisms or involvement in a world perceived as negative.

- *If a parent is reactive*—tending to react out of concern with his or her own feelings instead of calmly listening and taking in the child's communication—the child experiences being unreal or unimportant, and core development will be inhibited.

- *If a parent is depressed,* this too will naturally stunt the emergence of a child's healthy core, because a depressed parent is unable to make free and open contact with a child.

- *If the parent is a martyr,* always reminding the child—verbally or nonverbally—of the difficulty of parenting, the child will tend to shut down and not take the parent in.

- *If a parent is anxious and "stressed out"* the parent will turn inward, automatically projecting anxiety onto the child and the child's circumstances. This, in turn, can damage a child's sense of trust in himself and the world.

We cannot be perfect, of course, but all of us have a responsibility to be the best we can be. Having the courage to assess our parenting styles and try out new behaviors, adjusting our style for the sake of our families and ourselves, is a powerful step beyond A.D.D./A.D.H.D.

The Overparenting, Codependency Dragon

In many cases, particularly cases of A.D.H.D., the overparenting pattern of interaction with attention deficit children leads to a relationship of codependency. *Codependency is needing the validation of another person in order to gain self-validation.* People in a codependent relationship tend to be enmeshed, living without personal space. There's a parasitic quality to the relationship that repeats itself over and over, sucking each person unwittingly into a negative vortex. The end of this vortex is often a stormy eruption of negative energy.

When calm is restored after a storm or upset, there seems to be no ryhme or reason for the amount of emotion that was displayed. *The parent frequently vows never to get involved in that kind of behavior again, but invariably it recurs.* Once codependency is established, it takes on a life of its own, and neither person knows quite how he or she got there or how to get away. Unfortunately, the codependent dynamic is self-perpetuating.

Of course, no mother or father intends to create a codependent relationship with a child. In fact, *parents who fall into this trap tend to be highly conscientious and loving, with the very best of intentions.* However, as they enter the process of parenting, the personal history of the way they were parented unconsciously colors their interactions with their children. They (like all of us) automatically and naturally either fall into old patterns from the past or tend to parent in reaction to their own upbringing. Parenting hasn't been called the toughest job in the world for nothing!

Also, of course, parents have legitimate needs and stresses of their own that often conflict with their children's needs and stresses.

Fortunately, the process of sorting out the issues and soothing the stresses of parenting becomes easier once we as individuals and as parents strengthen our own inner core. We do this by forming the habit of touching base with ourselves, and respectfully honoring our inner feelings and needs.

With awareness, we can get out of our own way, which in turn helps clear the way for our children's core self to emerge. With awareness, the parenting problems disappear as we connect fully to the present moment, keep the long view in mind, and maintain our perspective. We lose the feelings of guilt and blame when we begin adjusting what is not working in our behavior and changing it. Soon we find that *awareness of our errors no longer contains any feeling of "ouch."* At that point, we are truly self-aware, at the beginning of true self-mastery.

Justin

Ten-year-old Justin exhibited codependent behavior with his mother and father, Karen and Sam, who centered their life around him. That is, they automatically paid more attention to his needs and feelings than their own. Karen, for instance, feared being rejected by Justin, was desperate for his approval, and paid all too much attention to him, while ignoring and neglecting her own needs.

This dynamic had begun at Justin's adoption, when Karen and Sam placed him at the center of their lives. When parents put a child at the center of their experience, constantly focusing their attention on the child while neglecting their own needs, in time, the parent–child relationship will become convoluted. It's as if the parties were constantly taking the wrong path in a maze and winding up in the same wrong place again.

Despite the fact that Justin and his parents loved each other very much, and that Karen and Sam's intention to be loving parents was of the highest caliber, their lives became emotionally wrapped around each other.

Consequently, there was no room for the parents to give attention to their personal lives, let alone to attend to their relationship, and no room for Justin to develop and grow as a separate, self-contained individual. As an only child, he was given a lot of toys, praise, and attention, while his real needs for independence, boundaries, and limits often went unrecognized.

Codependency involves a kind of parental overkill, in which the parent becomes overly identified and emotionally entangled with the child, losing perspective and objectivity. When the child gets a poor grade, for instance, the parent feels crushed. If the child has a disappointment with another child at school, for instance, the parent will not only keenly feel it but may actually show up at the school, in a futile and unrealistic attempt to protect the child from any pain.

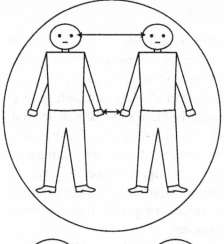

From Codependency
Stuck
Negative
Disembodied
Limited vision
Enmeshed
Hypervigilant
Controlling
Joined at the hip
No self-boundaries
Live in other's experience
Far from authentic self

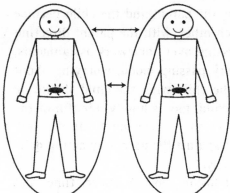

To Independent Individuals
Moving
Positive and proactive
Embodied
Focused
Effective
Confident
Takes risks
Free to be me
Self-contained
Lives in own experience
Connected to self
"I stand on my own two feet."

With my feet on the ground I can reach for the stars.

From psychostructural dynamics (PSD)

Add to this the frustration the parents feel deep within about never having (or more accurately, never making) time for themselves or their interests, and we have a potent mixture of unhappy feelings going around in the family. Because they were internally overwhelmed, frustrated, and unhappy, Justin's parents could not possibly model true self-respect and independence.

How can our children learn what we do not yet know for ourselves? *The answer is that they can't.*

Reacting Versus Responding

In a codependent parent–child relationship the parties are too close for comfort. The child's every move is scrutinized, and the parent tends to be overly watchful, usually waiting for something to go wrong. Instead of truly responding to a child, by quietly assessing what the child's needs may be, and exploring with the child, a lot of knee-jerk reacting goes on.

Reacting, in this case, means giving an impulsive response instead of a genuine, thoughtful one. A reactive response is not "clean," in that it is not based in the person's deeper intentions. Reactive responses create inner resentment and kill true communication.

In a codependent state, the parent and the child become overly vigilant toward each other, with the parent directing the child's every move, fussing over homework assignments, reacting to the child's every passing mood, worrying about the child, and doing for the child what the child should be doing independently. The child, too, is highly mindful of the power he or she holds over the codependent parents and, when frustrated, can use it against the parent by acting defiant, either openly or covertly.

Both child and parent become lost in space, time, and each other, caught in a repetitive pattern of behavior toward one another. This situation naturally creates a lot of anxiety for a youngster, effectively shutting down core development.

In codependency, a pattern soon emerges in which *emotional reaction becomes a substitution for healthy communication and interaction.* That's because we human beings are always looking for organization in order to be present and conscious. When we are enmeshed or codependent, we are literally organized around another person, and therefore are lost from ourselves.

The more children get pulled away from their own self-development, the harder it is for them to focus in a group situation. A child who has received too much parental attention and scrutiny can easily feel lost or at sea if an adult is not focused on him or her at every moment.

A.D.D. children may begin to fog out, constantly awaiting direction at school. A.D.H.D. children may act out negatively, becoming belligerent or oppositional as they express their frustration about the codependent corral they've been roped into.

The dynamics described so far occur in most families from time to time, but in the case of A.D.D./A.D.H.D.-identified children, they have been ongoing and constant, dominating the majority of the interactions between parent and child.

The Basis of Justin's A.D.H.D.

Let's examine how these dynamics played out in Justin's case, a typical A.D.D./A.D.H.D. experience.

Because Justin's core development was inadvertently being interfered with, he'd have frequent outbursts of anger that were really desperate cries of inner frustration. These outbursts perfectly mirrored his mother's and father's unacknowledged inner feelings of dependency, anger, and inadequacy. The unwitting projection of these feelings onto Justin contributed to his lack of self-security, which in turn was reflected in his inability to be "at home" even within the confines of his body.

In other words, Justin was getting to know himself through the unwittingly negative projections of his parents, instead of through positive self-discovery. His discomfort with himself was therefore laced with intolerable feelings of shame and inadequacy that resulted in low self-esteem.

When Karen felt anxious or incomplete inside, her energy would automatically go to Justin, who had become a kind of anchor for her emotions. This unwanted energy not only gave Justin undue and inappropriate control but also interrupted his process of learning to define himself realistically by accepting his limits as well as his potential. The inadvertent interference with the emergence of his core self was the underlying basis of Justin's attention deficit disorder. This pattern is typical in many families in which a child is identified with the disorder.

Codependency can shift only when one of the people chooses to re-form the relationship by learning to respect and maintain his or her own self-boundaries. The situation automatically transforms when a parent takes charge of his or her own life, the negative shadow self and the forward-moving, developing self.

When Justin's mother became involved with her ailing parents, Justin was asked how things were going. "Fine," he replied. "We're too busy to argue."

Storms

Just as an unstable weather system produces strong storms, the unseen frustrations and unmet needs of A.D.D./A.D.H.D. people and their families, coupled with their lack of physical grounding, often create dramatic, emotional outbursts. These off-kilter eruptions are out of all proportion to the situation at hand, leaving both child and parents feeling confused and bad about themselves.

Many times, parents, teachers, or spouses misread this "acting out" behavior as something deliberately planned to thwart them or make their lives miserable, when nothing could be further from the truth.

The outbursts can be so intense, the behavior so provocative, that it is hard for others not to be sucked into the vortex of negative behavior. If they are not alert to what's happening, others may even join in the negative energy, moving in and out of the space of the A.D.D./A.D.H.D. person, and coming down to that level. Research has shown that the interaction between A.D.D./A.D.H.D. children and their parents tends to be more negative than positive, creating a chicken-or-egg situation as both parties fall into negative patterns with each other.

Storms come about when both parties spin out their unorganized, unformed, needy selves, sometimes going to the extremes of violence, until the emotional angst plays itself out, changing the energy and making something different possible.

In nature, after a storm there's a sense of all being clear. Unfortunately, with people, storms often leave us feeling less than whole because we feel guilty and ashamed of our immature behavior. There goes one more little chunk of self-esteem, and the A.D.D./A.D.H.D. person becomes more anxious and less organized at the core.

In addition, because behavior tends to be ritualized and self-perpetuating, it becomes easier to fall into the negative loop as a habitual way of organizing and reacting.

Whenever we are in the presence of an emotional storm, we can be sure people have become disorganized within themselves; they are seeking some structure, even a negative one, to give form to their desperate feelings.

So what do you do when the storm is breaking loose? When children are "storming" with each other, it's best to calmly but firmly separate them. If you are a party in the interaction, try to extricate yourself as soon as possible and cool off. Walking away and taking a few slow, deep breaths will help you to pull yourself back to center.

It's sometimes too late when people are already engaged negatively, toe to toe. At those times we can only stop our own part of the upset and blow off the feelings of inadequacy as quickly as possible. The sooner we do an about-face and forgive ourselves, the sooner we will learn to conduct ourselves more positively next time. By stopping, and owning our participation in the negativity, while treating ourselves with compassion, we are also sending our children a powerful message of self-containment and safety. Later, when the storm has passed, we can reexamine the issues behind what happened.

The overriding goal is to become so aware and conscious of our own needs and others' that we don't get to the point of no return. Knowing the storm-warning signals is extremely important: when we are tired, hungry, stressed, and hassled, our primitive feelings naturally rise to the surface and erupt.

We can think back to our own childhoods, remembering how we felt when we were out of control, and what we needed. Using our own childhoods as a point of reference is a good idea, because it helps us to tune in to authentic childhood needs and perspective.

Lack of Embodiment

Justin's physical structure and use of space was typical for an A.D.D./A.D.H.D. child whose core self had not been given the space to emerge. For example, he had no boundaries and would move in and out of other people's spaces at whim.

At school, his lack of boundaries contributed to his habit of annoying his classmates. At home, in bed at night, he was terrified of being alone, because he felt disembodied (lacking ownership of himself) and unanchored. *When nobody else was around, Justin came up empty.* He had not had enough chances to experience himself, or enough time to be in his own experience of living. Justin felt like "no body." Sometimes, his body energy was fragmented, as if he were jumping out of his skin. His body reflected his inner chaos and disharmony.

The work on his PSD root points (explained in Chapter 4) was very powerful for Justin. As he connected to these key points on the body, he connected to himself and became more grounded. He began to own his body, his points of power, his space, and, ultimately, himself. This process was the beginning of his transformation.

Signs of Overparenting (Codependency)

While all parents tend to fall into codependent patterns from time to time, these dynamics tend to be dominant in families with A.D.H.D.-identified children. In order to move beyond attention deficit, it's important to examine and reform our interactions with our loved ones. Codependency must be eliminated if healthy boundaries and healthy interdependency are to be established.

The codependent parent typically:

- Gets overly involved in school projects

- Picks out clothes for the child

- Brushes the school-age child's hair

- Goads the child to get ready

- Has frequent arguments with child

- Directs social situations

- Can't bear to be separate from the child

- Constantly points out physical similarities of parent and child

- Neglects relationships with mate and friends

- Allows the child to sleep in the parental bed or sleeps in the child's bed

- Fears sending child who is old enough to overnight camp

The codependent child typically:

- Is fearful of or angry about separations from the parent

- Reacts to his or her teacher as if to a parent

- Has trouble going to sleep and waking up

- Wets the bed

- Is uncomfortable being alone in his or her room

- Needs parents to sit with him or her at homework time

- Needs help getting dressed

- Resists going to school

- Has few friends

Underparenting

On the opposite side of the need for parental balance is underparenting, a common dynamic in families in which children are identified with attention deficit disorder without hyperactivity. Underparenting can come as a result of a parent's work life, such as often working late or traveling on the job. Many such parents are highly successful individuals who have invested their energy in building their careers to the detriment of their children's deep, unseen needs for contact and connection. These parents may have inflated expectations about their children's achievements as well.

Another manifestation of underparenting is the parent who is at home but is always on the phone, cleaning, or otherwise not available to the children. The underparenter may also be in the grips of an addiction—to a substance, working, gambling, or shopping—or may be investing all of his or her emotional energy in a complicated love life, with little left over for the child.

Some underparenters have not faced the disappointments of their own childhood, or may be alienated or unconnected to their own inner core, making them unable to truly see their children.

Children who are underparented cannot develop a secure core because they are not getting the empathy and respect that a young person needs in order to grow. It's a lonely feeling to wait and wait for a parent too involved with other matters to give the young one sustained attention.

Both under- and overparenters tend to be deeply involved with themselves and with the images that they project in the world. They are usually individuals who have not had all of their essential needs met, so, sadly, they carry feelings of insecurity and discomfort deep within their own core, out of view to others.

Paul

Paul is a successful businessman and harried father who brought his eight-year-old A.D.H.D.-diagnosed son, Devon, in for treatment. While Devon met with the therapist, his younger sister, eighteen-month-old Anna was going to stay with her dad in the waiting room. Waving good-bye to his son, Paul seemed to struggle to stay awake on the couch. He fell into the sofa and "crashed."

During the day, Paul functions as an effective sales manager, leading a team of salespeople who also perform well. He's personable, positive, and tuned in to the needs of both his customers and staff. But when he gets home it's another story. With his family, he seems to be running on empty.

In the waiting room, his energetic toddler wanted attention. She wanted to explore. She wanted to relate. Paul obviously hadn't the energy for any of it. Sprawled on the sofa, he offered one negative directive after another: "Don't touch the magazines. Leave my shirt alone. Get the pacifier out of your mouth." Anna was becoming frustrated, and like all frustrated toddlers, her behavior became petulant and annoying. "Do you think she's going to have A.D.D., too?" he asked, only half in jest.

If one of Paul's clients were waiting with him, would he have been more present? We have the feeling he would have been. What makes a person with so much proven ability so powerless to organize himself with his own kids? It's as if there are two different people in Paul—the effective, positive sales manager and the ineffective, burnt-out dad. Why?

Paul is a good example of a phenomenon we often see in our society. It's happened to every parent—to me, to you, and all of us: we use ourselves up before we get to our children.

Paul seems blind to his need for some nurturing before he tends to his children. Instead of dealing with his authentic needs, or even being aware of them, he takes the path of least resistance: tuning out. He simply does not organize himself as a parent the way he does when he's out making a living.

When he comes home, all the pushing of himself that he did during the day grinds to a halt, and he seems to get stuck in himself. His body space shuts down, and his frame and structure no longer support his functioning.

Paul feels this as the need to crash. He feels overwhelmed. Consequently, he loses his perspective. When his children approach him, looking for contact, connection, consistency, and commitment, he gives out negative energy, treating them as if they were nuisances.

Let's back up and create another scenario for Paul. Suppose he still worked hard all day but treated his body better by eating more healthfully at lunch. Suppose he made physical activity a priority, finding the time to shoot baskets a few hours a week. This would eliminate some of the toxic sludge of negative emotional energy that builds up in anyone's life.

Suppose Paul allowed himself time to make a transition from home to work. He would leave the office with the knowledge that he was putting the workday behind him and would use the commuting time to get in a different mindset—that of a dad looking forward to enjoying his children.

He could picture himself enjoying his downtime, playing with the kids. . . .

If he were so tired that he couldn't function, a more centered Paul would have made other arrangements for Anna. If he were tolerably tired but still had to be with Anna, he could have washed his face and reminded himself to give her some positive attention. With a little up-front focus from Dad, Anna might have gone on to busy herself with the toddler toys available to her.

Maybe a more centered Paul would have taken the little girl for a stroll during their time together, or leafed through a magazine with her, or followed her focus to see what *she* found interesting. We can't know exactly what Paul needed to take care of himself—only he can know that—but we can be sure that if he were centered, he would have found a way to enjoy his time with his daughter despite his busy day.

The point is that we are not powerless over ourselves—even when we are tired—and there are lots of ways to meet our needs, and our children's. But we can find them only when we choose to tune in to ourselves and redesign what's going on.

This is intentional living. *You can create your life the way you want it to be, with unlimited energy available throughout the day, as long as you take the time to tune in to yourself.*

Signs of Underparenting

An individual caught in the underparenting trap typically

- Is habitually too exhausted to play with the child

- Utilizes an environment in the home such as an entertainment center in order to be away from the child

- Is not there, is traveling, or is unavailable to the child

- Gives in to the child's demands in order to avoid confrontations

- Allows an inappropriate amount of unsupervised behavior

The Good News

One piece of good news is that over- and underparenters can become balanced, relaxed, and more effective parents with a simple shift of *awareness*. Similarly, with this new awareness, adults who experienced out-of-balance parenting from their parents can instantly free themselves of these dynamics. *Awareness begins the turnaround process, and awareness is instant.*

More good news is that as adults, it's important to remember that we don't have to get the "C"s—contact, connection, consistency, comfort, containment, collaboration, constructive activity, and commitment—on schedule or exclusively from our parents. We can get them from any close, caring person: a relative, partner, therapist, teacher, or friend. At any age, the important process is needing them, getting them, having them, and ultimately, learning to provide them for ourselves, and others.

Breaking Free

Breaking free of the negative parenting patterns is easier than you may think. From a holistic perpective, the first and greatest principle applies: *start with yourself first.*

For the codependent parent it means taking stock of what is going on between you and your child, and looking for ways to increase your child's self-reliance. It's also helpful to back off when you are tempted to involve yourself in your child's experiences.

A Day in the Life of a Codependent Parent

7:30 A.M.

"Honey, it's time to get up. Come on, Sweetie, time to get up. Will you please get up now? Come on, it's getting late! You have to get up now! Why aren't you getting up! Do I have to pull that blanket off? Every day you pull the same stunt, and it's driving me crazy! Get up now, did you hear me? Get up! Get up! Right now!

4:00 P.M.

"Honey, you left the door open. Would you please shut it? What are you doing? Would you please take a minute to shut the door? And shut it every time when you come in, OK? Honey, you didn't shut the door yet. Hey! Where are you going? Did you hear me? I told you to shut the door! Come back here and shut the door! Just stop what you're doing and SHUT THE DAMNED DOOR!"

11:00 P.M.

"Listen, you have just got to go to sleep now! I already read you five stories! Remember what we said about lights out at 9:30? It's 11 o'clock! Why don't you just go to sleep? Why do you do this every night? No, enough stories! Do you know how sick and tired I am of your staying up so late every night? I'm tired and frustrated, do you understand? And you're driving me crazy! Oh, all right, all right—one page. But that's it! Then I really am shutting the light!"

For the underparenter, starting with yourself first means identifying the problem and then finding ways to nourish yourself before connecting to your child.

Take stock of your relationship with your mate, too. If it has suffered because of the energy you have invested in your child, or has overshadowed your child's needs, begin to think of ways to re-partner with your partner.

As you begin focusing on what you need in order to grow, you will naturally and automatically become more centered, grounded, embodied.

What a Parent Can Control

- His or her own feeling state
- His or her internal thoughts
- His or her actions
- The availability of certain food items
- The quality of toys, games, and projects available to the child
- The number of hours a child watches TV or plays video and computer games
- His or her vocal tone or quality of communication and connection between family members
- The consequences for violating family rules
- Young children's choice of friends
- Older children's privileges such as going to the movies or overnights
- Teenagers' use of the car keys

What a Parent Has No Control Over

- The child's feelings
- The child's attitude
- The child's opinions
- Older children's friendships
- Older teenagers' whereabouts

A Day in the Life of an Underparenter

7:00 A.M.

"Bye, honey. See you tonight."

5:30 P.M.

"Looks like I won't be home for dinner. We have a big project, and I have to finish it."

9:30 P.M.

"I am too exhausted to read to you tonight. See you in the morning."

What to Do When Your Child "Hurts" Your Feelings

1. Recognize that your feelings are hurt and that you are apt to be angry as well as hurting.
2. Buy yourself some time by choosing not to react with words or behavior until you've processed your feelings and thought the situation through.
3. Remind yourself that you can choose to keep the situation in perspective. There's more to your relationship with your child than the hurtful incident.
4. Love and care deeply for your child, but do so on a level that is unattached and maintains each person's independence as individuals.

One way to cut through old habits is to do less talking and more listening, less fussing and more connecting. When

What to Do When You Find Yourself in a Battle of Wills

1. Stop the battle and buy yourself some time by saying something such as, "I need to calm down. I don't want to fight with you."
2. Try to understand what your child wants on an emotional level.
3. Think back to your own childhood and how you felt at that age.
4. Be patient with the child's demands, and allow them full verbal expression.
5. Try to be as empathetic as possible without giving in to unreasonable demands.

Seven Commandments of A.D.D./A.D.H.D. Parenting

1. Honor your inner self.
2. Stay strong and calm in the face of immature behavior.
3. Be aware of your body, and take good care of it.
4. Take back your parental power, but do not attack.
5. Nurture your relationships with your partner/spouse/close friends as well as your children.
6. Have as much fun as possible.
7. Keep the long view in mind.

we listen on a deeper level, our loved ones feel more connected and better understood. The feeling that one is basically understood and accepted is the basis of healthy family life.

Control

The need to control others is a hallmark symptom of code-pendency. The importance of this dynamic in the development and maintenance of attention deficit disorder is noted even by Drs. Hallowell and Ratey, who favor a conventional, pharmaceutical approach to the disorder. In their classic work, *Driven to Distraction* (Simon and Schuster, 1994), they advise:

> Pay attention to boundaries and overcontrol within the family. . . . It is important that each member of the family know and feel that he or she is an individual and not always subject to the collective will of the family. In addition, the presence of A.D.D. in the family can so threaten parents' sense of control that they become little tyrants, fanatically insisting on control over all things all the time. *Such a hypercontrolling attitude raises the tension level within the family and makes everyone want to rebel. It also makes it difficult for family members to develop the sense of independence they need to have to function effectively outside the family.* (emphasis added)

Habit Thawing

Behavior, whether positive or negative, perpetuates itself. We human beings tend to repeat our actions and thoughts over and over. When our thoughts and actions are negative and unproductive, we easily become frozen and stuck in negativity. In that state, we want so much to be "right" that we may even forgo our own happiness.

When a child has the kinds of behavior problems associated with A.D.D. or A.D.H.D., it's easy for both parent and child to become stuck. The child does X, and the parents react with Y—even though the X–Y behaviors do not work for either one of them!

Moving beyond A.D.D. means changing habitual responses—*first* in yourself, *then* in the person carrying the
symptoms of A.D.D. By changing your own habitual
responses, you not only model growth and flexibility but also
catch the disorder off guard, so to speak.

Think of this process as like aikido or tai chi, the Chinese martial arts. In aikido, lack of resistance is used to overcome the enemy. When an attacker aggressively pushes
toward a person, the response is to step back, causing the
attacker to fall! Similarly, in tai chi, one's power comes from
being centered, balanced, and relaxed. In that state, an enemy
has little chance.

To encourage the formation of a strong, healthy core,
many new actions and behaviors have to be encouraged and
experimented with. The old negative patterns, the ones that
don't work, have to be ditched—no matter how comfortable,
habitual, or "right" they may seem to be.

Alex

*Ten-year-old Alex had become frozen in a negative, reactive state.
His impulses were so strong that he could not delay satisfaction
for a moment. If he was hungry, he had to eat immediately, even
if his family was in the process of fixing dinner. He would stride
to the refrigerator and help himself to whatever caught his eye.*

*Like many other children, Alex lobbied loudly and persistently
for material goods, but once he got them, he never seemed satisfied. His distraught mother described him as "going from one
obsession to another." One week it might be collecting the toys
issued around a certain movie character; another week it might
be collecting baseball cards.*

*Worst of all, when he didn't get what he wanted, he auto-
matically entered a state of negativity, rejecting any friendly
approach. Alex had a kind of arrogance, too, a quality that was
not appreciated by his teachers. Because of his lack of focus and*

attentiveness, the school authorities had suggested that Alex be referred to a pediatric neurologist. The neurologist diagnosed him as having A.D.D. and prescribed Cylert, an alternative to Ritalin.

Nevertheless, Alex's problems persisted, and soon he came to the Center for treatment. In the waiting room, it was easy to see that Alex was very attached to his mother. At first, he didn't want to enter the consultation room without her. His entire attitude was angry and defeated, and his self-esteem was close to his socks. (Later in our work together, he shared the fact that taking medication had made him feel worse about himself.)

Alone with the therapist, Alex was asked to define what the problem was. His explanation boiled down to: "I guess I just can't do anything right."

We talked about things he liked to do but didn't think he was good at, and he quickly mentioned playing ball in gym. "I never catch the ball. That's just the way it is."

His desire to be a better athlete was clearly a way into Alex's core self. That realization guided the following dialogue.

"Let's stop and look at this together, Alex. If you could choose to do it better, would you do that?"

This question caught his interest. "Sure," he replied, "but I can't."

"Let's see if I can help you get yourself out of the way. Suppose you did have the power to change: what would you do to become a better ballplayer?"

"Well . . . I could practice more."

"Yes. You could."

The look in Alex's eyes showed that a light had been switched on. He was beginning to grasp the concept that he did have the power to choose new actions.

"Alex, living is a lot like being in a car. Some people live as if they are in the backseat, with someone else driving. But others are in the front seat, driving the car themselves. If living your life was like being in a car, where would you be?"

"In the front seat, telling other people how to drive!" he answered with a smile. "Like when I drive my teachers and my *mom crazy by telling them everything I hate." Children have so much more perception into their own motivations than we grown-ups usually imagine!*

"But imagine how mueh more fun it would be to be the driver, and go where you want to go."

Any ten-year-old can understand this metaphor, and after that first session, Alex's self-awareness began to shift. He was forming a new consciousness about himself, and he soon began to realize that he had power to change his life. The next time we met, he proudly announced that he had begun

Handling a Temper Tantrum

The key to dealing with a temper tantrum is supporting yourself.

Here are some guidelines to remember the next time you find yourself in the presence of a full-blown temper attack.

1. Stay calm. Nothing gives a child more inappropriate power than an upset adult. By staying calm, you diffuse the situation and take the wind from the child's sails. You also model maturity for the child.

2. Change your body position. Place your feet firmly on the floor, straighten up, and take a couple of deep breaths. Placing your feet firmly on the floor and breathing deeply provides an opportunity to center and ground yourself before you take action.

3. Send yourself a supportive message, such as: "He's a child. He's having a temper tantrum, and I can handle this." Or, "Temper tantrums don't last long, I can deal with it." If there are critical people around, remind yourself that they have no power over you.

4. **If possible, leave the scene.** Tell your child you cannot communicate during a tantrum, and then leave! If your seven-year-old is yelling and screaming because you didn't buy her a toy or comb her hair "right," for instance, walk away until she calms down.
5. **Ride out the storm.** Children who try to control and manipulate their parents by having tantrums are just being immature and trying to get their way.
6. **If you cannot leave, give a warning and announce a consequence.** "You have one minute to end this tantrum. If you don't stop in a minute, you will not go to the movies on Saturday." Speak in as firm, but self-possessed a manner as possible.
7. **Never give in to a tantrum, no matter how tempted you may be!** Even if you decide to give the child what he or she wants, delay the gratification until the tantrum is over.
8. **Wait until the tantrum is over to talk to your child.** "You seem too upset to talk right now. When you calm down, we can talk."

practicing ball. He didn't realize it in these terms, of course, but Alex was empowering himself.

As he began making new choices and decisions, his frozen negative, reactive habits began to thaw. Within a month, he was ready to begin the process of eliminating the drug. His attentiveness and focus in school naturally improved, because he had a stronger self. Through simple body awareness and alignment exercises, he learned to connect to things outside himself. He was instructed to bang a tennis racket to reduce some of his pent-up anger, and thereby he gained awareness of himself, too. "I'm stronger than I thought," he said.

"Yes, and the anger you have will be very good fuel if you use it positively."

Alex's mother was thrilled with the new reports she got from school. As he became embodied, and tuned in to himself *as the creator of his own experience,* Alex was able to pay attention in a whole new way and give his teachers appropriate respect: his need to defiantly push against authority fell away. He was able to think and work more independently. Alex's defensive posture and negative habits seemed to melt away as the boy took charge of his attitudes and his life. Alex had effectively moved beyond A.D.D.

Coming Home to Chaos or Contentment

A difficult time for many parents of A.D.D./A.D.H.D.-identified children is after work. Plunging into a full evening of parenthood after a long day at work can be exhausting and disempowering. Parents may long for peace and relaxation in the evening, but instead find themselves coping with their children's incessant demands. This situation often leads to a buildup of tension, resulting in frustration and, finally, anger.

Renee is a nurse who tended to be tapped out at the end of her long workdays. Her husband, Mark, also was often fatigued after a full day working as an accountant, under a supervisor with a difficult personality. When the parents arrived home, one by one, exhausted after serving the needs of others all day, they'd be met at the door by nine-year-old, hyperactive Melody and her six-year-old brother, Greg.

The children would leap onto Mark, demanding piggyback rides. They'd grab onto Renee's legs, not even allowing her to take off her coat. Renee and Mark got into the habit of pushing the kids away, without realizing how rejecting their behavior was.

Worst of all, when the children didn't get the attention they craved, they competed with one another, squabbling and trying to make each other wrong. Instead of having relaxing evenings at home, enjoying their family, Renee and Mark were on edge and resentful more nights than not.

Mark tended to disappear in front of the TV after supper, and when Renee tried to catch up on the phone with a friend, the kids would still be clamoring for attention, with Melody often leading Greg in wild romps that resulted in noise, crying, and destruction.

These parents were torn between their desire to relax and "veg out," and their desire to be good parents. They both dreaded their evenings, often wishing that the other would do more of the work with the children and let them off the hook.

When Renee and Mark came to the Center, their family life was far from satisfying. The stress of putting up with Melody's hyperactive romps had put the couple over the edge, and each accused the other of contributing to the girl's problems. As they described the pattern of their evenings, it became obvious that, among other things, both Mark and Renee needed to redesign their evenings to provide themselves with more sustenance.

Redesigning their evenings meant creating a mental, and sometimes physical, transitional period that would help them make the adjustment from work to home life. Before she left work, Renee sat down and brought mental closure to her stressful workday. She went to the ladies room, washed her face, and used this pause in the action to tune in to herself and her needs, centering herself and grounding her energy. She used this time to think about her children in a positive way, using powerful affirmations based on the truth of her inner feelings and desires. *"I choose to enjoy my children tonight . . . I choose for it to be easy. . . ."*

For Mark, making a transition that met his needs involved using public transportation instead of driving to and from work. This enabled him to catnap on the way home, as he, too, mentally separated himself from his job and prepared to enjoy his children.

When they began consciously providing for their own needs in this transitional time, Mark and Renee found that their homecomings began to transform. When they walked through the door, they were ready to greet their children in a full and connected way. Mark found that, after changing out of his business suit, he actually enjoyed getting down on the floor and playing with the kids.

Because the parents were paying more attention to their own needs, they were better able to support each other, too. Instead of bickering about whose turn it was to be with the children, they decided to take turns. Renee found that better utilization of her answering machine kept obtrusive phone calls from interrupting her evening. When she wanted to initiate a call, she did it at a time when Mark was with the kids.

With Mark and Renee more relaxed, the kids relaxed more, too. Since they were each receiving better attention from their parents, they began playing with one another in a more positive way as well.

Focusing on your personal needs has a rippling effect, like a stone cast into water. As one person empowers him- or herself in a healthy way, each family member is inspired to do the same.

By attending to your own needs, you are modeling centered behavior in an authentic way that will have a positive

Why People Resist Going for Therapy

1. I'm not crazy. In past generations, psychotherapy was associated with mental illness. This is no longer the case, of course, but old beliefs die hard. Therapy in our time is often focused on growth and development.

Let's face it: we live in a stressful, fast-paced world. Taking an hour a week to tune in to our inner selves and what we need for peace of mind and contentment is a very sane and healthy thing to do!

2. My child (or spouse) has the problem, not me. Your child may be carrying the bulk of the symptoms, but if you are living with an A.D.D. person of any age, you have a problem, too. Your child or spouse may need one-on-one therapy sessions of his or her own, but each member of the family needs support and insight into their particular needs, too. A.D.D. affects everyone in the family. When there is movement away from the disorder, everyone will benefit enormously.

3. I'd like to go for therapy, but I can't afford it. The question that follows, then, is, how can you realistically not afford it? What price do you put on peace of mind—your own, your child's, and the rest of your family's?

Even if you don't have a lot of money, there are clinics and therapists who will work with you. If you are short on funds, have fewer sessions—nevertheless, each session you attend should have long-lasting helpful results.

Somehow we all manage to come up with the money when the car needs repair, but we hate spending it on soul or psyche repair. The trouble is that we are then in danger of going through life chugging along, spewing out the smoke of negativity and victimization instead of cruising down the highway, in control of ourselves and going where we really want to go! The truth is that therapy with a competent professional is one of the best investments you can make for yourself and your family.

impact on your family. You will also be displacing your child's negative symptoms as the modus operandi of the family, and putting yourself and your needs back in their rightful place— at the center of your life, where your true power lies.

There is no more inspiring example for an A.D.D./ A.D.H.D.-identified child than a parent who is truly at peace with him- or herself and living life on a higher, more purposeful, positive, and conscious level. And there is no better weapon against the disorder itself than a calm, focused, self-empowered parent.

The Importance of Therapy

Families living with the problems connected to A.D.D. need help. That, of course, is what this book is all about, and why it includes exercises and ideas designed to get the process of recovery in motion.

Simply reading the book will give you new information and ideas about attention deficit disorder and how to handle its symptoms. That is useful, but reading the book *plus* actively *doing* the exercises greatly increases your progress. That's because the exercises operate on a level deeper than the verbal level.

In addition to this book and others on the market, *psychotherapy* or *counseling* can help families struggling with A.D.D.

What to Look For in a Good Therapist

Therapists don't have the answers—not good ones, that is. Instead of telling you what to do, a good therapist will guide you to finding your own internal answers. He or she will help by clarifying, supporting, and even challenging old beliefs when necessary.

Shop around for a licensed therapist or counselor. Remember, you are paying, and you have a right to good service. Scheduling appointments or speaking on the phone with a couple of different professionals will give you an idea of who they are and how they work.

There are many different schools of therapy and theories about how people grow and change, but social research consistently finds that the single most important indicator of success in therapy is the bond between the particular therapist and client.

Here are some of the basic qualities to look for in a therapist:

A good therapist will treat you, and every member of the family, with respect at all times.

A good therapist will be warm, kind, and nonjudgmental.

A good therapist will help you to clarify your personal issues, and not "take sides" during personal conflicts.

A good therapist will be trustworthy and open in his or her communications.

A good therapist will challenge your beliefs as necessary.

4

Step-by-Step Recovery

*The moment one definitely commits oneself, then
providence moves, too. Whatever you can do, or dream
you can do, begin it now.*

Goethe

*I have discovered that no one who learns to know
himself remains just what he was before.*

Thomas Mann

This chapter offers an overview of the eight major steps that
lead to a full and lasting recovery from A.D.D./A.D.H.D. Also
included is a detailed list of tools and techniques designed to
help you make the shift from disorder to centered, grounded
living.

As with the stories of others who have successfully made
this journey, the hope and expectation is that these key concepts will inform, instruct, and inspire you to greater understanding so you can move away from the dynamics of A.D.D./
A.D.H.D. *When the basic principles that underlie recovery are
thoroughly understood, they move from the realm of theory into
the realm of everyday life where positive change can take place.*

The opportunity in the crisis of A.D.D./A.D.H.D. is a large
one: it is the chance to renew and rejuvenate your life expe-

rience, to rework and revitalize every detail of living so that you will be more self-aware, self-accepting, and empowered. The light at the end of the A.D.D./A.D.H.D. tunnel is beautifully bright, peaceful, and luminous.

Moving Beyond A.D.D.: What It Takes

The path beyond A.D.D./A.D.H.D. is comprised of specific actions and attitudes that can be undertaken by anyone who is willing to begin with himself or herself. By noticing and taking charge of your inner life, you will be off to a strong start.

You can expect positive results when you put these ideas into action and allow them to shift your consciousness, but bear in mind that there is no magic wand that will make every negative symptom disappear instantly. Recovery from A.D.D./A.D.H.D. is a gradual process; the positive aspect is that *gradual change is lasting change.*

Step 1: Decide to Move Beyond A.D.D./A.D.H.D.

This first, all-important step opens up healing power by allowing new ideas, attitudes, and behaviors to emerge and take root. These in turn break the rigidity of the person's feelings, attitudes, and thoughts about A.D.D./A.D.H.D.

Making the decision to move beyond A.D.D./A.D.H.D. means taking a stand against any hopeless feelings or unnecessarily negative thoughts about the disorder. When people make a firm decision to free themselves from the disorder, movement naturally and automatically occurs because the disorder is no longer given the upper hand. Instead, recovery and healing become the focus of attention.

Think for a moment about two typical smokers who say they wish to free themselves of the smoking habit. Smokers who constantly tell themselves that stopping is impossible or extremely difficult, or that it will involve too much sacrifice, will not succeed in quitting. Their focus is on the difficulty of the task, and their attitude is laced with negativity. On the other hand, smokers who make a firm decision to quit will try all kinds of new behaviors until they reach their goal. These new ideas and strategies empower them by providing the persistence necessary to make the shift in consciousness that is necessary for quitting.

Similarly, a firm decision to leave attention deficit disorder behind frees energy and creativity. When Carol's doctor told her that her son, nine-year-old Josh, had symptoms of A.D.H.D. she felt bereft, depressed, and hopeless. Part of her was angry with Josh for being a difficult child, and part of her was upset because she felt that the disorder was a negative reflection on her family life.

To comfort herself, Carol accepted the explanation that A.D.D. was a physical problem based in Josh's brain.

From this perspective, Ritalin could help control the symptoms, but the attention deficit was something Josh and his family would have to live with for the rest of their lives.

This discouraging point of view robbed Carol, Josh, and the rest of the family of true happiness. In her heart, Carol found Josh's attention deficit hard to bear.

Only when she met Myra, a mother who had taken a drug-free approach to treatment for her son, did Carol's perspective change. Myra was in the process of effectively moving beyond A.D.D./A.D.H.D., and when she shared information about the process she inspired hope in Carol. Carol made a firm decision to try a new approach to the disorder, too. "I decided to free Josh, and myself, of course, from A.D.D. *no matter what it took*," she told us later. "Not only that, I started seeing getting past A.D.D. as a kind of adventure."

An incredible amount of energy was released as Carol reexamined every facet of her life and Josh's to find the clues that would make recovery possible. Instead of thinking that A.D.D. was something with which she and her loved ones had to live, she put her focus on finding solutions. By laying her discouragement down, Carol found that many new ideas, attitudes, and behaviors surfaced and took shape. Josh's recovery did not occur in a straight line, of course, but when he became negative Carol was able to step back and detach from the negativity and get her focus back on center.

After about a year of sticking with the firm decision to move beyond the disorder, Carol found a checklist of symptoms that she had originally written down, and went through them one by one. To her delight, Josh no longer met the profile of a person with A.D.D. His development was back on track, and her relationship with him was more comfortable than ever.

Step 2: Start with Yourself

It is vital that you begin using the principles and ideas in this book in *your own life first* before introducing them into the lives of your children.

"Do as I say, not as I do" is a sure way to fail in our efforts as parents. In this book, for instance, you will find information about how to become centered and grounded; these deceptively simple ideas cannot be bestowed in mere words, however. They need to be experienced, practiced, and, finally, mastered before they can have the desired powerful effect.

When six-year-old Seth was running amok in a hyperactive frenzy, his anxious grandmother, who had been recently introduced to the concepts of centering and grounding, shouted, "Seth, you calm down now! Ground yourself!" Seth laughed and continued spinning out of control. Her message was nothing more than an empty phrase because his grandmother was herself uncentered and ungrounded!

In order to effectively use these ideas with children, the adult in charge must have mastered them on an *experiential* level. Seth's mother, Jane, who was further along in the process, was able to shift her son's behavior when she arrived on the scene. That's because Jane dealt with herself first. Seeing Seth spinning out of control, she first reminded herself that his off-kilter behavior was not malicious, insane, or evil; he was simply a little boy who did not yet know how to organize his energy.

She placed both of her feet firmly on the ground and took a slow, deep, relaxing breath before speaking to him. When she was ready, she delivered the same message to him that his grandmother had, but this time the words were backed up by Jane's own centered, grounded power. The message got through to him on a level that was far deeper than mere words.

Step 3: Learn to Center Yourself

Learning to center yourself is a key component to recovery from attention deficit disorder. By *centering*, we mean *living in the authenticity of one's own personal experience.*

In order to center yourself, you need to know yourself on a deep, intuitive level, "inside and out." Making a realistic but positive assessment of yourself and your life is a good place to start. (You'll need to clearly identify your personal strengths, your basic needs, what gives you pleasure, and what causes you pain, and become keenly aware of the activities and behaviors that infuse your life with meaning and vitality.) Sitting down and making an inventory of all these factors is a good way to gain the relaxed self-awareness of who you are at the core.

The goal here is not to find your center and stay there forever and ever, however. We all must live life on its own terms, and this means that we will frequently be pulled off center. Instead of thinking of your center as something solid and fixed, think of it as a balancing mechanism, one that your actions, thoughts, perceptions, and attitudes need to calibrate to or harmonize with.

In pottery, a lump of clay has to be centered before it can be shaped into a useful object. So, too, the process of centering ourselves is the *beginning* of the process of becoming ourselves, not the *end*.

As an example, consider a mother who is reading a book while her children play with friends in the backyard on a sunny day. The mother is in the middle of an exciting chapter when the children approach her because they want ice cream. They begin to plead with her to drive them to the store.

The mother with little awareness of her basic need to be relaxed will give in to their pleading—in other words, she will be pulled off center. She'll put the book down and drive the kids to the ice-cream shop, possibly resenting it all the way. Later, she may even blow up at the children for something else that happens because she is unconsciously angry about placing their needs before her own.

The mother who is centered, or learning to be centered, will assess the situation differently. When approached about driving the children, her first internal question will be something like, "Where am *I* about this? What are my needs in this situation?" Because she is in the middle of an exciting chapter she will put off their request, perhaps suggesting a different game for them until she is ready to take them someplace.

Her answer to the children, even if it is, "Not now," will come from the center of her own self-awareness. Because she is in tune with herself on an authentic and fundamental level, the children will tend to comply with her response, too. When we are in the presence of someone who is centered, we intuitively sense the person's power.

Step 4: Learn to Ground Yourself

Your body provides valuable clues about your authentic inner state and is also a powerful instrument of change. Learning to read the signals of your body and literally re-form yourself when you feel disempowered is another important step in the process of recovering from A.D.D./A.D.H.D.

Think of yourself for a moment as an energy system, and you will see that energy is expressed in the very way you move and form your body. Every moment of every day, waking or sleeping, the living structural system of your body organizes, disorganizes, and reorganizes itself. Mastering the way we form and shape our body makes a profound difference in the way we think and feel as we move along, experiencing life.

The energy of A.D.D./A.D.H.D.-identified individuals is disorganized, ungrounded, and uncomposed. They lack a grounded sense of what's going on inside and tend to be unconscious about the way they occupy their space. Consequently, their energy is not fully available to them and they cannot focus on a positive goal.

The anxiety, confusion, and inner insecurity of A.D.D./A.D.H.D.-identified people have interfered with their natural development, and this is often reflected in the misalignment of different parts of the person's body. The head may go off in one direction and the neck in another, for instance. Similarly, the arms and legs seem to shoot off every which way, and there is a subtle but definite lack of firm footing when the person stands, walks, or runs. Once development is back on track (when the person receives appropriate amounts of the "C" factors), bringing the body into alignment will facilitate better use of the person's natural energy. The energy can now be used for self-discovery, positive exploration, skill building, accomplishment, or fun.

Of course, no one can bring another person's body into alignment, but as adults we can model a different way of carrying ourselves in balanced alignment for our children. When we form and shape our body in a way that helps us to sustain our own positive energy, our children will unconsciously imitate this mastery in time.

Also as adults it is essential that we begin to read the signals of our own and other people's bodies if we are to have the knowledge and sensitivity to overcome A.D.D. We can notice if we are slouched over and ask ourselves what that is about so that we can deal with the thought or feeling that is literally "pulling us down." We can pull ourselves into better alignment before we make even a small decision. We can notice our children's use of body space and gain important clues about their authentic inner feelings and needs.

When Barry noticed that his A.D.D.-identified son was slouched in a chair staring into space, he took the boy's body formation as a clue. Instead of sending a critical message, such as, "Why are you just sitting there staring?" he asked his son, "Is something making you sad?"

When Keith had trouble focusing on his homework, his mother shared her experience of finding better focus when both feet were firmly on the floor. "I do better when I pull myself together, like this," she said, demonstrating for him. She then exited the room, leaving him to his work. "When I came back later, he was sitting up straight, working," she told us. Keith accepted his mother's technique because it came from her authentic experience and not as a bossy directive.

Step 5: Honor Yourself, Including Your Shadow Self

Honoring oneself and one's shadow means facing, respecting, and examining one's feelings, even the most uncomfortable ones, and accepting oneself at a very deep level. When we honor ourselves we naturally and automatically honor the other people in our lives, too, because honor and judgment cannot exist in the same space.

By making a decision to honor and even cherish ourselves at a deep internal level, we wisely do away with the critical judging voice inside that will tear us down at every turn if we let it. Instead, we give ourselves, even the unseen part of ourselves, the gift of validation and acceptance. By honoring the totality of who we are, including our lesser impulses, we move toward true self-understanding. While it is not always possible to understand ourselves in any given moment, it is vital that we try, and we can be sure that our efforts will be rewarded in time.

Every human being has a dark side, a shadow side that produces thoughts and feelings of which he or she may not be proud. When we reject ourselves by disrespecting this aspect of ourselves, or trying to shut it away, we are actually cutting off an important source of information about our innermost needs. Just as we need to learn to read our bodies, and the way we shape our energy, we also need to "read" the needs that our shadow self is signaling. Honoring ourselves at the deepest level is a giant step to getting in the right relationship to ourselves.

Nora was bothered by her twelve-year-old daughter, Beth, who seemed ungrateful for all Nora did for her, from the gifts she purchased to the rides she provided. She often found herself thinking of Beth as a "little ingrate" and sometimes experienced an intense feeling of what she could only describe as "hatred" toward her daughter, a feeling that was intolerable to Nora.

Before Nora undertook the challenge of moving her daughter beyond A.D.D., she'd feel guilty and upset about having these negative feelings toward her daughter (whom she adored at heart). When these feelings would arise in her, she would attempt to ward them off by doubling her efforts to please Beth. She'd purchase new, better, and different toys and styles of clothes, and provide more services in the hope that Beth would respond positively. The results of Nora's efforts were disappointing, however; Beth seemed even more ungrateful, which meant more frustration for Nora.

After Nora made a decision to honor herself, even her shadow side, the picture changed dramatically. In the light of self-honor, she was able to look at her unpleasant feelings more closely.

"I thought Beth was hateful and ungrateful because I had made myself her slave!" she later told us. "I gave her all sorts of stuff and never got anything for myself. Making her happy had become my main project in life, and of course, that didn't work. Deep inside I was unhappy about all that giving."

Nora stopped making clothing purchases for Beth and instead spent some money revamping her own wardrobe. Instead of looking for toys and games for Beth, she began indulging her own healthy pleasures. Instead of driving Beth all over town, she encouraged her daughter to make other arrangements when it was inconvenient for Nora to jump into the car to take her someplace.

The inner feeling of resentment toward her daughter became a window through which Nora was able to identify her own needs. When Nora's behavior changed, so did Beth's because she discovered a new respect for her mother. Nora and Beth were now free to enjoy a more positive relationship with each other.

Step 6: Establish Healthy Boundaries

A healthy boundary is the acknowledgment that we are separate and distinct individuals with separate and distinct realms. It is the notion that I am me and you are you, and that my thoughts, ideas, feelings, responses, and experiences belong to me, and yours belong to you.

Establishing healthy boundaries with our children can be difficult because children start out as dependent babies. It is right that we bathe, feed, and carefully watch our babies when they are tiny, but from toddlers on, children really do need for us to back off and let them experience life for themselves.

Barbara is doing an outstanding job of parenting her two-year-old daughter, Hana. When asked for the secret of her success, she replied, "I know when to get out of the way and let her happen."

Knowing when to get out of the way is a very important skill, particularly in parenting A.D.D./A.D.H.D.-identified children, for it allows young people to experience life for themselves, which leads to self-discovery and the formation of a core identity. Children need time to follow their own noses, just as adults do. They need time to get to know themselves without a parent hovering over or prompting them. They also need a certain amount of authority over their own lives. The wise parent, for instance, will not argue with a clothing choice, because clothing the body falls into the child's realm, not the parent's.

When Trina received a rabbit for her birthday she was thrilled, but her joy faded when her mother rushed to the hutch ahead of her so that she could show off the new pet to Trina's friends. When Trina came home to find that the rabbit had already been fed and his cage cleaned, her sense of ownership was further diminished. Whenever Trina mentioned the rabbit, her mother would go get it, hold it, and stroke it. In the end, the mother completely took over the experience of having the rabbit and even criticized Trina in front of others for not taking care of it! Trina was left feeling sulky and confused, her self-esteem lowered by the whole experience.

Trina's mother had not respected a boundary. The rabbit was given to Trina, not her, and the job of caring for the pet also belonged to the girl. Had she been allowed to fulfill her responsibilities, Trina would have gained valuable self-esteem and self-respect. Instead, she was robbed of the opportunity to bond with and care for her new pet.

Of course, mothers are not the only space invaders. Fathers, too, can inadvertently step across these personal boundaries.

When eight-year-old Ron expressed an interest in joining Little League, Brian, his father, signed on as an assistant coach. This action was not necessarily an invasion of Ron's boundary, of course, but the way Brian functioned as a coach was. Brian insisted on moving Ron into the position he wanted to play, often arguing with the head coach in the process, and sharing information that Ron had told him privately at home.

During the games, Brian hovered over Ron and focused on him to the exclusion of all the other players, embarrassing his son as a result. At home, Brian adamantly insisted that they practice every evening after supper, even when Ron would have preferred to play with a friend.

By the end of the season, Ron's interest in playing baseball was low, and Brian was annoyed and dismayed. He thought he was being a committed father and doing "what dads are supposed to do." He did not recognize that his actions around Ron's baseball experience were invasive.

Brian's lack of awareness in this area is all too common. It's easy for parents to fall into the trap of unconsciously thinking that we "own" our children and have the right to invade their territory, and therefore to lose our objective distance. Only by making a commitment to recognize and maintain healthy boundaries will we be able to step back and get out of the way as our children learn to discover life for themselves—not us.

Fortunately for Ron and Brian, the story had a happy ending. When he entered into the recovery process, Brian began maintaining and respecting his boundaries with others, including his son. The next year when he coached in Little League, he treated Ron like just another member of the team, and consequently, the two had a more enjoyable season.

Step 7: Take the Long View

Your relationship with the A.D.D./A.D.H.D.-identified person in your life (or with yourself, as an adult with attention deficit) is going to last a lifetime and go far beyond A.D.D./A.D.H.D. During recovery, you have to bear in mind that moments seared with emotional intensity are just that—

moments. Keeping the long view in mind will help you to keep any transitional situations or leftover negative or unproductive behavior in perspective.

When Sharon and Jake stopped allowing ten-year-old Andy to have soda pop and potato chips on school days, Andy hit the roof. He tried every form of manipulation to get his parents to change back to the old ways, but Sharon and Jake were able to hold firm because they could see farther than their son: they took the long view of Andy's well-being and therefore were able to remain both calm and strong in the face of his childish protests.

To heighten your awareness of the long view, it's helpful to remind yourself to occasionally lift your eyes and literally to look out into the distance (as suggested in the tools and techniques section that follows). Using your eyes in this way will help strengthen your ability to keep the long view in mind on both the symbolic and real levels.

Step 8: Practice

Make frequent use of the self-tuning tools and techniques explored in this book, in the following section and elsewhere. They will help you to master the basic concepts of recovery from A.D.D./A.D.H.D. dynamics.

Self-Tuning Tools and Techniques

Imagine that you are being given a little black bag to fill with useful skills, actions, and exercises to help you move beyond A.D.D./A.D.H.D. Each of the items in the imaginary bag is readily available and easy to carry out. Some are well known, while others are special techniques developed as part of the psychostructural dynamic (PSD) program discussed earlier. All of them raise the level of energy and promote centering, grounding, self-honor, and the establishment of healthy self-boundaries.

Tuning A.D.D./A.D.H.D. Systems

A.D.D. Goal:
Get energy moving within—completing self-circuit

- Organize self-feedback from "I am not" to "I am"
- Own your own space—start to stand on own two feet—sense and focus personal power
- Use breathing to clarify intention—take action

A.D.H.D. Goal:
Slow down, contain energy

- Pause, breathe
- Hold on to yourself—stay in your own space
- Exercise your eyes: keep head still/move eyes
- Establish calm, quiet mind: become embodied—connect PSD root points
- Use breathing to slow system—focus attention on breathing, practice deep breathing while lying down, or in simple yoga

These deceptively simple self-tuning techniques work like a pebble cast into a body of water; they have a powerful ripple effect that brings positive change to a person's entire life experience. We have found them to be very effective at the Center, and they can easily be adapted for use at home.

They are:

Direct Communication

Proper Breathing

Still Point (a calm, quiet mind)

PSD Root Points

PSD Jet Knees

Eye Focusing

"Groking"

Toning

Letting Go of Anger

Witnessing the Self

Contacting the Higher Self

Visualization

Use of Art to Find Out

Opening the Heart

Each is described in the following pages.

Direct Communication

The basic idea that needs to be communicated is that there is nothing "wrong" with the A.D.D./A.D.H.D.-identified person, and that it is in that person's power to overcome the negative symptoms of A.D.D./A.D.H.D.

Even a young child can understand a statement such as, "You have a lot of energy—that's good. But you need to use it better." Other useful statements include: "Growing up is learning to take care of yourself." "The power lies in you." "You are good, but what you're doing right now isn't. What can you do instead?" "If you want things to be better, you've got to make them better." And let's not forget those all-time powerful parental words, "I trust you to find a good solution," and "You can do it."

Proper Breathing

We cannot overemphasize the importance of deep, full breathing because *breathing is the point at which life, mind, body, emotion, and energy all connect.* The breath is the interface of the mind and body.

Not many people would dispute the fact that breathing patterns reflect emotions. Everyone has at some time gasped in fear, sobbed in grief, guffawed in laughter, or experienced the deep, trembling breath of anger.

But the relationship extends beyond this, for *a change in the breathing pattern can also alter an emotional state.* In a state of deep relaxation in which breathing is deep, full, and easy, for instance, it is virtually impossible to feel fear. It follows, then, that *using the breath to re-form ourselves is perhaps the most powerful action we can take to alleviate stress on a mind, body, or energy level.*

Deep breathing is also vital for effective brain functioning, as it helps supply oxygen and necessary nutrients to the brain. One of the most powerful tools of recovery, breathing allows enhanced receptivity to new perspectives and other changes in thought and behavior.

Deep breathing is based in what the Japanese call the Hara, the source of personal power. To breathe properly, relax and allow your body to align itself into a comfortable (not rigid) position. Then pull in a slow breath through your nose to the Hara point (see the discussion under "PSD Root Points"). If you are breathing properly, your chest and torso will not rise—they will expand outward. Breathe out through parted lips. Do this frequently throughout the day, whenever you are in a stressful situation, or to increase alertness. The time it takes to breathe also provides a moment in which we can take a reflective pause. Stopping the action allows us to reassess any situation so that we can proceed with more intention and intelligence.

Finding Still Point: Creating a Calm, Quiet Mind

This simple exercise promotes inner peace, calm, and quiet, which in turn promote more positive and focused living.

Get comfortable in a chair, resting your arms on the arms of the chair, or your hands on your thighs. Breathe deeply and slowly, and allow your mind to settle down. Close your eyes as if closing a door that keeps you securely inside. Sense your stillness and wholeness. Imagine that your breath is sending a golden glow of peace to every part inside you. Let your mind rest.

This still point is available to all of us at any time of the day or night, but it can easily be lost in the rush of life. Once you have practiced locating your still point you will soon find it instantly available to you just by thinking about it. Finding your still point is empowering at any time but can be a lifesaver during times of stress or strain.

PSD Root Points

There are key points on the human body that help a person to self-organize. In psychostructural dynamics they are called "root points." These *root points are both real and symbolic;* they can be understood by young children as well as adults.

The master point is the Hara, or Source of Energy, located an inch under the navel. This is the place where breath emanates. Other root points are:

1. Feet, our foundation and base, which connect us and ground us to the flow of gravity

2. Solar plexis—the self-centering point

3. Chest and heart—the home of core feelings

4. Shoulders—that shape us to withstand life challenges

5. Throat, connecting head to body, giving the power of expression

6. Eyes, "windows of the soul," the ultimate two-way mirror

7. Crown, the top of the head, the powerful organization station

PSD Seven Root Points

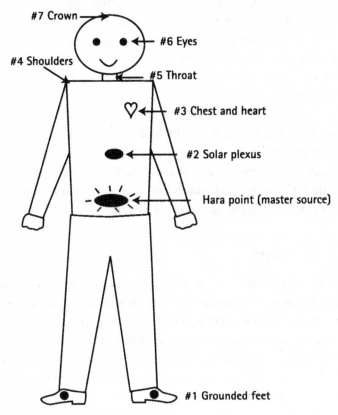

From psychostructural dynamics (PSD)

Taking a few moments to touch base with them as explained in the following section—and really *own* them—is a start on the lifelong road to self-empowerment. (Note: Soothing, rhythmic background music enhances the experience.)

Sit in a straight-backed chair, place your feet securely on the ground, and find your inner quiet space. Allow your head to lift at the crown, as if it were lightening up or floating.

Take a relaxed breath through the nose, drawing in from the Hara point. Think, "I own my body and the power of my body."

As you continue breathing, focus on each root point, and the power that the point contains. As you breathe out through gently parted lips, sense each point of your body, as if your breath were sending awareness into it. Appreciate the powers of each root point.

Send a breath to your feet and really feel your feet, their size and shape, and the way they connect you to the ground. Imagine roots growing from your feet, going deep into the earth. Sense your connection to the ground.

Send your breath and concentration to the solar plexus, sensing the energy and power of that root point. Make contact with your center.

After each breath, go back to the Hara to draw the next breath, and send the energy of your breathing back to each point in a circuit.

Send your breath to your heart, your very core, and seat of your deepest emotions. Let your heart relax and open as your chest expands. Imagine that the deep, calming breath is like a powerful light entering your heart and chest.

Allow your concentration to move to your shoulders, a root point of your self-structure and strength. Notice how your shoulders feel. Are they slumped, rounded, or tight? Make an adjustment by balancing your shoulders and widening them.

Move your breath and concentration upward to the throat and neck. This is a critical point because many people, especially those affected by A.D.D./A.D.H.D., are cut off from connecting their head to their body at this place. Breathe into your throat, focusing on its power to help you express yourself appropriately and assertively. Think of your head and neck connecting to your body, helping you to fulfill your intentions.

Let your breath and attention focus on your eyes and face, relaxing them, and tuning in to your power to take the long view as you fearlessly face the issues of your life.

Finally, move your breath and awareness to the crown of the head, the station of power and self-organization. Imagine useful energy coming in through the top of your head as your forehead muscles relax. Let your head rise freely at the crown.

As you continue to breathe, send the vitalizing energy of your attention and your breath in a complete circuit of these vital root points.

The symbolic, yet real, action of acknowledging your root points helps you to claim ownership of your self and your power.

PSD Jet Knees: Tuning In for Alignment and Present-Moment Focusing

Working as a school social worker in an inner-city school, I (Rita) developed this exercise to help children to focus. It's called Jet Knees because when I was shopping in an upstate mall, I saw a large crowd gather around a raised stage as two men sat, signing autographs. I asked what was going on and was told that they were members of the New York Jets football team. Here were two men in a tip-top physical and mental state. They were successful and seemed to be enjoying themselves at that moment.

I noticed how they were sitting, and to my amazement they were in the exact position of the exercises I had done with my students! From that moment on, the exercise was called Jet Knees. The kids loved hearing this story, which helped them to identify the exercise to a sense of power.

Try Jet Knees when you are sitting at a desk at work or at home to bring yourself into better alignment.

Start, as always, with a deep, full breath and distribute it slowly throughout your body. Move forward to the edge

PSD Jet Knees: Establishing Self-Control

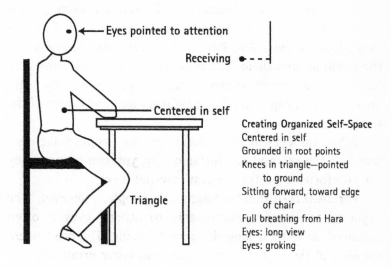

Eyes pointed to attention

Receiving

Centered in self

Creating Organized Self-Space
Centered in self
Grounded in root points
Knees in triangle—pointed
to ground
Sitting forward, toward edge
of chair
Full breathing from Hara
Eyes: long view
Eyes: groking

Triangle

From psychostructural dynamics (PSD)

of your seat, sending your knees downward so that a triangle is created in the lower half of your body. You will notice that your head comes forward, and your breath will deepen automatically. Your upper body will be in better alignment from head to toe. Once grounded, look up and out, to a point in the horizon.

By grounding the body energy, Jet Knees quiets the mind, enhances the breathing process, and allows you to be more fully present and aware. This in turn frees energy, making it available to focus, persevere, and stay on task effectively.

Eye Focusing

Human eyes have been called the windows of the soul, and wisely so. On a physical level, the optic nerve is close to both the thinking part of the brain (the cortex) and the more primitive feeling part (the limbic system). A large portion of the thinking and feeling we do regarding life experiences comes through our eyes.

The eyes of an emotionally stable, self-accepting person are dynamic but calm. They are able to move in all directions, looking close and far, as they seek, search, and sense the world around them. Someone with a strong, healthy core has eyes that reflect security and self-possession. Eyes are open, curious, eager to take in information, and aware of the long view.

When the eyes of emotionally healthy people make contact in a relaxed and comfortable way, you can be sure they are comfortable on the deepest internal level.

For A.D.D./A.D.H.D.-diagnosed people, however, the capacity to connect comfortably to others' eyes is often impaired, as is their long-distance focusing. The head is not stable, and therefore the eyes dart and move erratically.

To experience the way an A.D.H.D. person "sees" life, lift your eyes from the book for a moment, and move your eyes and head in all directions as you try to think about something simple and concrete, such as the names of the capitals of the states. You'll find that clear thinking is practically impossible when your head is not anchored and your eyes are not still!

People with the symptoms of A.D.D./A.D.H.D. tend to lock their vision in a certain range, too. (TV viewing has a part to play in this problem because it, too, locks the eyes in an unnaturally short, two-dimensional range. See Chapter 8.) Because they see parts, and not the whole, their thinking and perception of reality is distorted. The eyes of an A.D.H.D.-identified person tend to dart frantically, while the eyes of the A.D.D.-identified person are frozen.

To experience the frozen state of A.D.D., hold your gaze in one place for a very long moment. Then turn your head slowly, asking yourself what you missed seeing while in the frozen position. The answer will be, "a lot"!

The common description of A.D.D.-identified people as "foggy," and A.D.H.D.-identified people as "wild" is partially due to our subconscious perception of their faulty eye contact and range limitations. Their anxiety and internal disorganization are mirrored in the way they use their eyes.

"Groking" or Expanding Outward

"Groking" is a science-fiction word that means "becoming one, or merging, with something outside yourself." When you "grok" you open up and connect, taking in and giving out energy and awareness at the same time.

In this exercise we practice sending our energy to a specific point outside ourselves. The reason is that when the inner space is chaotic, a person cannot perceive the outer world accurately; only when we calm our bodies and quiet our minds can we truly receive an outer experience.

First, ground and align yourself, breathe deeply, and then turn your attention outward, letting your eyes settle on an object in the distance. Allow yourself to connect fully to this object, giving it your full attention and awareness. Because you have connected with yourself first, you can now have the energy available to perceive the object accurately.

Children are fond of this exercise, which helps them to tune in and connect on a deeper level. This prepares the way for increased focus and enhanced connection with the world outside yourself.

Toning

Hearing the sounds that one can make can be empowering and energizing; sounding off can often move a person off a "stuck" position. At the Center we tell children to try "toning" when they are bogged down or stuck in their homework or other tasks: they are encouraged to go to a place where they will be alone and make sounds that range from very high to very low. This often shifts their experience, freeing them to go back to their work.

Three Steps to Focus

Step 1

To open up a child's range of vision, start by noticing your own range. Take a moment to think about what it's like to be at the ocean's edge, gazing far out over the sea. Or perhaps you prefer to imagine yourself atop a mountain, viewing distant trees. The action of looking out over the long view is relaxing for our eyes and opens us up on a deep, internal level.

Ask yourself: Do your own eyes get enough "play," focusing on things both near and far? Whose eyes do yours connect with? What was eye contact like with your own parents in the past? Were your parents' eyes warm and inviting, or cold and critical? How wide is the lens of your eyes? Notice your peripheral vision.

Step 2

Without "doing" anything about it, notice the degree of eye contact that your child displays over a period of a week or so. A child with severe A.D.D. symptoms can actually avoid direct, sustained, relaxed eye contact with others for days at a time! Notice the times he or she does make contact, as well as when contact is avoided. If the child's eyes tend to shoot in every direction, bouncing off the walls, notice that, too.

Step 3

Begin to quietly bring your new awareness to everyday circumstances. When you greet the child after a separation, for instance, casually try to "catch" his or her eyes and smile. Social scientists have found that what happens in the first four seconds of contact actually predicts an entire day's encounter between two people! Making sure a person carrying the symptoms of A.D.D. gets a warm, relaxed hello, with direct eye contact, is a small behavior that has big impact and payoff. If you use baby-sitters, share this knowledge with them, too.

Another important action to take is scanning distant sights with your child for a few moments each week. Look out the window, for instance, and say, "I see a bird, far away in one of those trees! Do you see it, too?" Gazing into the distance is very helpful in restoring a full range of motion in the eyes. You can say, "I just noticed a squirrel on the roof of that house way over there. What do you notice?" Looking into the distance both symbolically and literally helps us to keep things in perspective, and to be receptive to our experience outside ourselves.

Around the house, point out objects across the room. If the child has chosen a meaningful poster to hang in his or her room, for instance, you might say, "I like to look at that picture of the boat. I like the way the water sparkles."

A walk in the park, woods, or other natural setting is wonderful for eye focus, because it gives the eyes an opportunity to take in things both near and far.

You can also talk to your child directly about his or her eye movements, if you keep the tone of your communication light. Children enjoy testing their peripheral vision, for instance. You might say, "I'm going to hold this pillow by the back of your head and bring it around front. You look ahead, and tell me when you can see it from the corner of your eye."

Letting Go of Anger

Anger is an energy that must be released. Very importantly, it is also a signal that the person is not in the right relationship to him- or herself. If not released in a safe and productive manner it will be released destructively, or turned inward, causing depression. Every home needs an area or instrument whereby family members can release angry feelings.

At the Center we use a tennis racket to beat a large pillow placed on the couch. A punching bag or sandbag would also be appropriate for the release of anger. Our clients often report creative new solutions for this task, such as the woman who "strangles" towels, the teenager who throws ice cubes into the bathtub, and the dad who schedules time to hit a pailful of golfballs, each one representing a frustrating person or situation in his life!

Witnessing Yourself

When you step back from your immediate experiences, noticing what is going on outside and inside, it's like opening a window and letting in fresh air. This powerful witnessing technique will help restore inner balance, putting you in a better position to take positive action. The first step of witnessing is to emotionally detach and notice what is going on around you and how you are reacting to it, as if you were a friendly but impersonal observer. If your child is out of sorts and acting immaturely, being a witness will help restore your sense of perspective. During this process, make inside comments such as "I'm so annoyed that my stomach is in knots and it's all over an unmade bed."

Being a witness of your own thoughts, feelings, and behaviors helps you to become more aware and consequently to become a powerful agent of change in your life. As a witness, you will consistently touch base with the power you have to make more positive choices for yourself.

Meeting Your Higher Self

Tune in to yourself by breathing deeply, closing your eyes, and going within. Complete a self-circuit from the crown to the feet. Imagine you are standing in a place you love on a beautiful day under a brilliant blue sky. You are standing with your feet planted firmly on the ground, anchored to the center of the earth.

As you become rooted in your own space, pretend that you see a figure walking toward you. As the figure gets closer, it looks at you with warm, loving eyes. Imagine that the figure's eyes connect to your eyes on a deep and true energy level. As the figure moves closer, its energy expands toward you, filling you with a warm, loving glow. You realize that you are experiencing your higher self.

The higher self is a symbolic representation of you at your very most alive and focused best. Imagine that you learn the name of this figure and befriend it. If your system of beliefs allows, you can call on this symbolic person when you are in need of guidance or feel you've lost the way.

Visualization

Visualization is an important tool for creating positive life experiences. It consists of simply thinking about, imagining, or "seeing" something positive in your mind's eye. When we visualize, we focus our energies on creating good feelings and positive experiences.

For instance, parents who are traveling back home after a long day at work can see themselves entering the house, enjoying the greetings of their children, changing clothes, and then playing with the kids. Similarly, parents who take a moment out of their busy workday to "see" their children, relaxed and smiling, in their mind's eyes are setting the stage for a more positive future experience.

Imagine your child doing the tasks you would want him or her to do, imagine the family having fun together, imagine yourself enjoying your day to the utmost. These pleasant visions not only soothe and calm the mind but also seem to have an uncanny effect on our thoughts and behaviors.

Use of Art to Expand Awareness

Art is a medium that reveals what's going on below the words, deep within. To do this exercise, you'll need paper and drawing materials. Before reading the rest of this section, draw and/or have your loved one draw (on separate pieces of paper) a person, a tree, a house, and a family. The drawings should be done in a spirit of spontaneity and freedom. When you are done, use the witness technique to find out more about your inner world.

The completed drawings provide other valuable clues about the artist's sense of self. They are unconscious self-portraits.

As you analyze the drawing of the figure, ask yourself: Is this person large or small? Does the body include hands, which represent the power to do for oneself, or not? Is the expression on the face happy or sad? Note the size of arms, hands, and fingers, which symbolize our ability to grasp control of ourselves. Does the person look anchored, or as if floating in space? Does he or she have eyes, nose, ears, and mouth to take in the world around? Is the picture balanced or off-kilter?

The drawing of the tree and house also represent the person on a deep, unconscious level. A tree with birds in the treetop and many colorful leaves is a picture of healthy and dynamic mental energy. On the other hand, a person who draws a shriveled tree trunk with a deep hole is providing a clue about a formerly traumatic incident in his or her life, and the emptiness that person feels within.

When looking at the drawing of the tree, ask yourself: Did the person who did the drawing connect the tree to the earth, or is it floating? Is the trunk strong and secure looking, or frail and weak? Is there detail and definition in the upper part of the tree, or is the crown of the tree absent of leaves or internally empty? Let your intuition help you explore the meaning in the picture.

When analyzing the drawing of the house, look for openings to the house that represent the ways in to the person. (One A.D.D.-identified boy drew a home with no door or windows!) How large is the house? What, if anything, is outside the house? Is there a path connecting the house to the larger world?

Similarly, the portrait of the family, especially one drawn within a circle, reveals a lot about the person's experience in his or her own family. Where are the people placed in relation to each other? Who is the largest figure? Where is the child in relation to the other members of the family?

Also note the confidence level of the person while drawing. Does he or she seem comfortable? Cross-outs and erasures can be indicators of anxiety or fear.

Save the drawings for comparison after several months of centering, grounding, and learning to sense the inner self. You will be amazed at the difference in the drawings when the symptoms of A.D.D./A.D.H.D. have diminished.

Open Your Heart

This last simple but powerful exercise can be done anyplace, at any time. Simply draw in a few full breaths through your nostrils, exhaling softly through your lips, while telling yourself inwardly, "I am the center of my experience. I am valuable and strong, and I now open my heart to everything good in myself."

The power of this exercise lies in its ability to raise consciousness, strengthen self-esteem, and focus awareness on the positive aspects and perceptions of our self-experience.

This sampler has given you some examples of how to tune in to yourself and strengthen your inner experience as you move along the path that leads beyond A.D.D./A.D.H.D.

You will find that becoming a centered, grounded, self-accepting individual is literally a breath, thought, and behavior away. The more you live from your center, in touch and in tune with your needs, the better a role model you will be for your A.D.D./A.D.H.D.-identified loved one, helping him or her to find inner calm, too.

5

Parent Empowerment

Love is the commitment to nurture your inner growth.
Until you make this commitment, no relationship will
be fulfilling enough to carry you through its trials and
turmoils.

Amrit Desai

Father, you cannot teach your boy to be a man—you
must be one yourself.

Folk saying

For the parent dealing with a child who exhibits symptoms of A.D.D./A.D.H.D, lasting change begins with the process of self-empowerment, because *only an empowered parent can struggle with the disorder and win.*

By parent empowerment, we mean tuning in to your fundamental needs as a unique individual, being aware of what they are, and allowing them to be expressed day to day.

The good news is that when you begin to empower yourself, you automatically and concurrently unleash powerful internal forces, such as *clarity, resolve, intuition, and creativity*—forces with which you may have lost touch along the way. Just as the exhausted star of an action/adventure film seems to summon up strength from an unseen source at the

very moment he or she most needs it, the process of empowerment will put you in touch with these resources and others that have been lying dormant within you all along.

As you actively encourage yourself to transform the
negative effects of the disorder into self-awareness, self-
acceptance, and strength, every scrap of energy, every fiber
of your character will be tested, and every asset utilized. But
*could there be a more important undertaking than saving your
child from a disability that, if not overcome, will bring the
child, and the rest of the family, years of misery?*

Parents who meet the challenge of empowering themselves and help their youngsters to move beyond A.D.D.
experience themselves and their family life as more whole,
healthier, and happier than they had ever imagined. These
courageous women and men did nothing more than what you
can do, and they all started where you must start—within
yourself. By identifying and satisfying their core needs, they
put themselves in the right relationship to their innermost
selves, and learned to accept and trust their instincts on the
deepest level of being.

Once the empowerment process was under way, they used
their newly discovered inner resources to begin moving away
from the chaos and negativity of the disorder moment to
moment. Soon, you too will learn to move through the day
more and more easily, calming, focusing, and strengthening
your A.D.D./A.D.H.D.-identified child, yourself, or your
spouse. Doing so, you will be creating the conditions that
allow for the emergence of the authentic core self.

At the end of the process, not only will you have your
child or mate back from the grip of the disorder, but you will
have an enhanced relationship with yourself, too. In the process of initiating the recovery from A.D.D., you will have
become a calmer, more focused, and more positive individual, one who has developed the ability to sustain a positive
outlook and actions even under stress.

This is the hidden gift inside the crisis of A.D.D./A.D.H.D., and it's a reward that anyone coping with the insidious symptoms of the disorder richly deserves.

Forgive Yourself

Setting the stage for your empowerment means clearing the deck of any guilt and regret about past events.

As parents, and as people, we've *all* made mistakes, even awful ones. Maybe you hired the baby-sitter from hell, or yelled at your children for spilling something. Or hovered over them. Or picked on them because you were tired. What parents haven't fought in front of the kids, or allowed too many sweets or violent video games? Because you are a highly conscientious parent, you may harbor unpleasant feelings and even sometimes secretly wonder if your mistakes were the cause of your child's A.D.D.

The truth is, *nobody*, not even a powerful figure such as a parent, "causes" a person to "get" A.D.D./A.D.H.D. The derailment of development that we call A.D.D./A.D.H.D. involves many aspects of living and many influences.

If you are carrying unproductive, negative feelings about past parenting mistakes, *it's time to let them go.* Here's an exercise to free you *forever*:

Make a list of every parenting error you have ever made, as far back as you remember. If you beat yourself up for those mistakes, be sure to include that on the list, too!

Tell yourself you are going to feel bad about these mistakes just one more time—*the last time ever.* Go over the list, feel the sting of regret if you must, and then go on to ask yourself: What useful lesson did I get from this particular mistake?

Once you have identified the learning, write it next to, over, or under the mistake. Cross out the mistake, and underline the lesson.

Then smile and tell yourself, loud and clear, *I fully forgive myself for these and any other mistakes. From now on, I choose to live in the present, the only place of empowered action.*

If self-blame for past events comes into your mind again, as it probably will until new habits are formed, remind yourself that the statute of limitations is in effect and let it go! Thoughts and feelings about past mistakes only weaken us as parents and rob us of the energy we need to be in charge.

Putting Yourself First

It is ironic that the first step to becoming a committed and heroic parent, one strong enough to grapple with A.D.D. and win, is to become *more self-centered.*

Until we learn to organize our day-to-day lives around providing ourselves with a positive outlook, healthy pleasures, and whatever else we need to feel comfortable and powerful, attention deficit disorder will have the upper hand.

Putting your personal needs first is an elusive but obvious first step to displacing A.D.D. and, ultimately, eliminating it from your child's life.

Selflessly giving to an A.D.D./A.D.H.D.-identified person, catering to his or her needs *while ignoring your own,* is a prescription for disaster. Yet, many conscientious parents are so busy meeting the needs of the A.D.D.-identified child, their other children, and their spouse, boss, coworkers, friends, and parents that their own core needs have gone too long unseen, unheard, and unmet. That is a lonely and unsupported—and ultimately intolerable—place to be.

None of us can be an effective parent when we're exhausted, frazzled, or enmeshed with the disorder's impulsive or fuzzy negativity. In that disempowered state, the parent's whole life becomes a reaction to the disorder, as the parent selflessly organizes his or her entire life around the child's "happiness." *We cannot make anyone else happy—we do not have that power.* We can only happily be in the right relationship to ourselves.

Hoping to satisfy the child's desires for the latest toys and games, trying to arrange the household, and sometimes the whole world, for the benefit of the child can create a situation in which the adult's mood tends to swing up and down with the child's A.D.D. symptoms and behavior. Parents who engage in this misguided approach are unknowingly putting their children at the very center of their own lives, *where they themselves should be.*

A flight attendant demonstrating the proper use of an oxygen dispenser in case of an accident instructs passengers to take care of themselves first, before assisting the children traveling with them, and the same goes for helping your A.D.D.-identified child. You simply cannot be an effective parent when you are discouraged and out of touch with that which brings you joy and increases your vitality. Grinding yourself down will not raise up your A.D.D./A.D.H.D.-identified child—but empowering yourself, by making some of your own needs primary, *will.*

It's sad to think that many people live their entire lives without giving much thought at all to their personal needs. Growing up, they were the good and compliant children who met the expectations and needs of their parents. In school, they obediently tended to their work, meeting the agendas of their teachers. In adult life, they focus on being responsible to their spouse, family, and superiors at work.

There's nothing wrong with being responsible, of course, but we pay far too dear a price for it when we leave our innermost selves out of the process of our lives.

Upside-Down World

In a fast-paced world where false needs are ceaselessly promoted through the media, our true needs are often unseen and ignored. In a world where both parents often hold down jobs, as we busily fulfill our responsibilities to others, we can fail to even realize we are neglecting our inner core self.

Providing ourselves with whatever we require for growth, pleasure, and vitality becomes the very *last* item on our busy agendas—*the one that there's no time for*—instead of the *first*. No wonder the world seems upside down!

The Empowerment Process

Empowering yourself means boosting your energy by taking the time to identify what your particular body, mind, and spirit require to make life joyful and worth living, each and every day. It means creating some time just for yourself, alone and away from work *and* family. It also means sorting out the differences between our true, inner needs and the ubiquitous false ones promoted by the media.

Empowerment means providing for ourselves while knowing what we need from others, and being able to comfortably ask for it.

Remember that as parents, we are models not by what we say, but by *how we live*. Taking the time to focus on our own core, meeting our deepest needs (maybe for the first time in our lives), by calming and strengthening our sense of purpose on the inside, at our center, is the most important step we can take—for ourselves and our A.D.D./A.D.H.D.-identified child.

How to Identify Your Needs

Primary needs are needs that can be met only on the inside. To get started identifying your particular primary needs, ask yourself, "What do I need that only I can provide for myself, on the inside?" To meet the need, ask yourself, "How can I satisfy this need in my everyday life?"

Here's a list of potential needs to spark your thinking process. We suggest you choose no more than one primary need at a time to get the empowerment process started:

- To take care of my body

- To be calm inside

- To feel worthwhile

- To live in harmony with my true values

- To accept myself

- To have fun

- To appreciate my life

- To make a positive contribution

- To enjoy what is beautiful

Primary Needs of the Body

Psychological needs are tailored individually, but the needs of the human body are more of a one-size-fits-all kind. Every body needs exercise, both aerobic and weight-bearing, as well as healthy food, such as fruits, vegetables, and whole grains, and adequate rest. Providing your body with what it needs day to day is empowering; *ignoring your physical needs is disempowering.*

If you tend to neglect or ignore your physical needs, it's time to think about changing some basic health habits—not by berating yourself, but by supporting yourself, little by little, to replace unhealthy habits with healthy ones.

By slaying the dragon of hypocrisy, you'll also become a powerful model for your children as they form their health habits, too.

He Who Walks Uprightly, Walks Securely

Which comes first, the posture or the attitude? Like the eternal riddle of the chicken or the egg, our posture and attitude do a kind of mutual back-and-forth dance, affecting how we feel. Studies indicate that depressed people can temporarily lift their spirits by smiling, for instance.

Think about times when you are feeling calm and confident, happily living out of a sense of your true inner priorities. How do you hold your body?

Your head lifts effortlessly from the very top, stretching your neck comfortably, and your shoulders naturally widen, allowing greater intake of breath. Your face relaxes. Your back lengthens and straightens, and your feet feel firmly planted and balanced on the ground. If you are very happy and peaceful, when you move, you move with grace, almost as if floating through space.

If you are in need of a quick mood enhancer, try adopting this positive posture, and you will find that the term *pick-me-up* has a literal counterpart in the physical world—one you can use at any moment of the day.

What Do *You* Need?

When we speak of human needs, the first things that come to mind for most people are food, shelter, and clothing. Many overworked, overstressed, and emotionally unsupported parents, when asked about their personal needs, throw up their hands in confusion. "I have everything I need!" they reply. "I have a place to live, enough food, and clothes."

These parents have confused survival needs with living needs. Their needs are being met, but only on a survival level, and *they are not even aware that their deep personal needs are going hungry.* Real living far surpasses survival; it involves the satisfaction of deeper, more primary, and individualized needs.

Nancy

Nancy was an overstressed, overworked mother whose six-year-old son, Jason, had symptoms of A.D.H.D. Nancy's husband was often out of the house or away on business, leaving the household and the overseeing of the children's education in Nancy's care.

Nancy performed admirably. She arrived at work on time and fulfilled her job responsibilities to her supervisor's satisfaction, even if it meant skipping lunch hours and breaks. She did all the household shopping, paid the bills, prepared food, arranged play dates, even involved herself at Jason's school as a volunteer in order to ingratiate herself with the staff, in case Jason needed extra attention.

In short, she was a diligent wife and mother—with one unfortunate trait: in her attempt to handle her myriad responsibilities, Nancy habitually focused 100% on others, and left herself out of her own life. Like many other overworked, conscientious parents, she tended to overparent Jason, by trying to meet his every need.

Naturally, this was impossible, and Nancy found herself more and more overwhelmed, less self-contained, and less self-centered and grounded. Her children, too, particularly Jason, followed suit, growing in an uncontained, ungrounded way.

As he became more and more riddled with the symptoms of attention deficit, his negative behavior became a habit that was constantly repeated. Nancy, who was trying to meet his needs, was sucked into the vortex of his out-of-control, negative energy, and life became miserable for the two of them.

Only when Nancy took the time to identify and attend to her own needs did the tide turn.

As a young woman, for instance, she had loved to sing. Her fantasies about her future always involved music in one way or another, and singing gave her enormous pleasure. But after Nancy had established a nonmusical career, married, and had kids, her love of music lay like a forgotten toy and was eventually packed away in the attic of her unconscious mind.

As a responsible grown-up, Nancy had concluded that she had "no time" for music. At first she missed singing, but after some years, she seemed to forget all about it. Even the enjoyable fantasies faded from her thoughts as her life got caught up in the daily grind.

For Nancy, singing and music became an unmet need. Deep inside, that unmet need was robbing her of personal joy. Upon learning that an old college chum had cut a CD, for instance, she found herself becoming uncharacteristically jealous.

When Nancy identified her deep inner need for music, and gave herself permission to find a way to incorporate it in her present-moment living, her spirits began to rise and come alive. Music energized her and strengthened her at the core.

She started searching for special music to enjoy on her commute to and from work. Then she joined a community singing group that met weekly and gave performances a couple of times a year.

Though Jason battled her on some nights before she left for rehearsals, in time he seemed to accept and respect her need to do something for herself. When her group gave a performance, her family was in the audience, cheering.

At home, she began dealing with Jason and her other children from a place of greater internal authority. With her vitality enhanced, her posture and vocal tones reflected more conviction when she needed to discipline the children.

As his mother's core strengthened, Jason was less able to manipulate her with his negative symptoms. He responded to the change in the way she felt and how she was delivering her power to him. From a simple "look," that connected them in a firm but loving way, he picked up on the expression of authority coming from her eyes. The more self-empowered she became, the more she could detach from his negativity, while still providing what he needed.

Nancy grew able to remain self-contained and self-possessed, even in the face of Jason's irritating behavior. She began disciplining him from an internal reserve of love and strength, guid-

ing him to seek his own best interests with cooperative behavior. He responded to the conviction and clarity of her position, and gradually, his symptoms abated.

Identifying her need for music and meeting it was only one of many steps Nancy took to empower herself, of course, but it was one of the most important ones.

Music put her in touch with a pleasure and process that was hers alone. It freed her from her daily concerns and made her more relaxed, whole, and centered. By filling her with pleasure, her involvement with music empowered her at her core.

If you seriously want to free your child, yourself, and your family from A.D.D./A.D.H.D., we urge you to take the time to reflect on these challenging questions now:

What are the unmet needs in *your* life?

What has become of your dreams? Are they being nourished or starved?

What symbolic message can you send yourself that reverberates deep inside, reminding you that you are a person standing separate from house, home, job, children, and spouse?

How will you express your right to be fulfilled in a way that allows you to have daily, ongoing pleasure and positive energy at your very core?

Authentic Inner Needs Versus False External Needs

If you find yourself craving material goods when you think about your inner needs, you may be in the grip of a false need. False needs sound like this in our minds: *If I only had a . . . I'd be happy.*

But don't worry. False needs can be good clues to your more authentic inner needs. So instead of trying to extinguish your material desire, think about what it may represent as a symbol for a primary need.

For example, wanting a vacation house may symbolize a need for more free time, or for an expanded view of oneself. The desire for glamorous clothing or jewelry may stand for a need to be more special. A car may represent greater freedom, a house may stand for more security, and wanting a new sound system may equate to the desire for enhanced self-expression. Let your imagination help you find the meaning behind your wish.

Freeing Your Inner Child

OK, we admit that the term *inner child* has been a little overused, but the idea that we all have an unformed child inside us is useful for those dealing with the effects of A.D.D.

Living with the negative effects of the disorder can cause people to shove their inner child off into the corner so that they can get through the day, coping. Consequently, *the child-like part of the personality, the part that needs fun and pleasure, becomes sulky and resentful. And the adult may not even realize what has happened. All he simply knows is that he feels distressed, or shut down!*

The goal of parent empowerment is not to outgrow the inner child, but rather to find a way to meet its needs. When our inner child is healthy and whole, it brings a sense of freedom, joy, and delight to our days. When you are more in touch with your healthy inner child, you will still be a responsible adult—you'll just get more fun out of life!

Before your inner child can be truly free, however, you will need to tune in to the immature parts of your personality. This part, too, needs to be known, accepted, and understood in order for you to identify your authentic needs and desires.

No Perfect People

There are no perfect people, no perfect parents, and certainly no perfect childhoods. Remember, one of the basic themes of

One-Minute Empowerment Exercises

1. Take a deep breath, or several deep breaths. Remind yourself, "I can be strong and calm."
2. Silently choose to accept your A.D.D./A.D.H.D.-identified child just as the child is that very moment—whatever he or she is doing—even if it's slurping cereal. You'll deal with the challenges later; right now, just send silent love and support.
3. Anticipate pleasure. Wherever you are, whatever you're doing, stop for a moment and notice the pleasure available. Ask yourself, "What's nice about now?" If you are standing in a bookstore reading, do you love bookstores? Do you like the way they smell? Do you feel good about sampling books, and learning and growing? Let the pleasure of good moments sink into your core.
4. Pause during the day to close your eyes, breathe deeply, and touch base with a feeling of gratitude for the good in your life. It's always there, waiting to be acknowledged and experienced.

a holistic approach is "no blame and no guilt." *Blame and guilt, like perfection, have no place in a positive mind-set.*

There is simply nothing "wrong" with your child or yourself—you are wonderful people who are growing and developing! In the spirit of adventure, you are becoming an empowered change agent, noticing what works and what doesn't.

Part of this empowerment process requires looking back at the way you were parented so that you can be more aware of yourself in the present moment. If you are like everyone else in the human race, you are probably carrying a few notions about life, or about yourself, leftover from childhood, that just aren't useful anymore. When we go back and clean up our past, by *releasing any leftover bad feelings, putting the past in perspective, and understanding it*, we are really giving ourselves the gift of empowerment. The old limitations fall away, and we feel a surge of fresh energy to help us meet our present challenges.

The Way Out Is the Way Through

Unfortunately, the shadow of unmet needs of childhood does not fade away, even if it does fade out of everyday awareness. Until we pull our buried lonely, ashamed, hurt, or angry feelings out by the roots, they have a way of reaching up and robbing us of the flexibility, freedom, and joy that a healthy inner child could be bringing to our adult lives.

We revisit the past not in order to see ourselves as victims but rather to empower ourselves to break free of old, outgrown, or faulty points of view about who we are, and who we can be.

A person who is courageous enough to search through the deficits of his or her own childhood will find not only muck in need of cleaning up but also treasure ready to be recovered. Taking the time to compassionately review your early life will yield rewards that will empower you as a person and as a parent—rewards great enough to help you free your child from the clutches of A.D.D.

Notice and Accept

As an experiment, tell yourself you're simply going to observe your inner state of being for a few days. Do this by making frequent spot checks on your inner self. At various moments, pause to ask yourself, "What am I feeling? What do I need in order to make this a more positive moment?"

Allow yourself to notice and experience any negative feelings *without acting on them*. Used this way, negative feelings help to guide us to what we need to do. Once the feeling has been fully experienced it will automatically transform to usable energy. Noticing and accepting is a tool that allows you to mobilize yourself in a positive way so you can be in charge of yourself again.

How Were You Parented?

When we lack awareness of how our parents' parenting style affected us, we can end up repeating their mistakes without intending to. The way we were parented is in our "hard wiring"—it's what we think parenting is. That's fine—if we had perfect parents. But since we didn't, it's useful to take some time to think about the positive and negative ways your parents interacted with you. That way, the positive aspects of their parenting can be kept, and the negative ones chucked.

This process may seem obvious, but how many of us actually take the time to sit down and clarify these issues?

Parenting in Reaction

Another danger we face if we don't take a hard look at our past is *parenting in reaction to how we were parented.* This kind of parenting is disempowering because it is not a truly free choice. In our attempt to avoid our parents' mistakes, we may tip the scales out of balance by choosing the opposite, equally inappropriate behaviors.

Mary Beth

Mary Beth had a critical mother who never complimented her or praised her in any way. Because of this, as a child, Mary Beth often felt lonely and unloved. She longed for the parental attention and affection that seldom, if ever, came her way. Naturally, Mary Beth's self-esteem tended to be low, despite her considerable achievements in the world and an unceasing commitment to "perfection."

Her marriage to Warren, who was highly attracted and deeply committed to her, was a step toward healing, but it did not transform the problem. Since no one can change another's insides, Warren's affection could not fully extinguish the pain of Mary Beth's unexplored inner needs. Because these needs were still going unmet, she tended to focus on what she wasn't getting from him. If Warren neglected to praise her for something she thought praiseworthy, such as making an especially tasty dinner, she felt his silence as an inner sting. It did not occur to her to praise herself, nor would she ask for what she needed unless her resentment reached the boiling point.

When their son Jonathan was born, Mary Beth vowed that things would be different. Her child would be praised and complimented as she had never been. Jonathan's good looks and sunny nature made praise-giving easy for Mary Beth. His every coo, smile, and scribble became cause for celebration. Mary Beth's praise of Jonathan and everything he did was unceasing and reached every aspect of his life. Her adoring eyes searched endlessly for something to praise and compliment in her young son.

Unfortunately, however, Mary Beth's inner dialogue with herself was far different. Inside her heart, the echoes of her mother's criticisms were still resounding, loud and clear.

When anyone close to her was unhappy, she unconsciously (and sometimes consciously) blamed herself for some failing in the relationship. When Jonathan was diagnosed with A.D.D., she felt sure the disorder had been caused by some failure on her part. In short, internal criticisms ruled her inner world, even as she kept up a steady stream of compliments for her son.

By the time Jonathan was eight, he could be described as a "praise junkie." If his teacher did not actively praise every dotted i and crossed t he would become sulky and resentful. At home, he demanded a full-tilt celebration every time he did anything as incidental as throwing a tissue in the wastebasket. And ironically, because children reflect their parents' deepest inner attitudes, Jonathan's self-esteem was as shaky as his mother's, despite his large appetite for praise!

Mary Beth had made an understandable error as a parent: without realizing it, she was parenting in reaction to her parents' parenting styles. Only when she truly, deeply, and authentically empowered herself, by facing her unmet childhood needs and meeting them on the inside, could she free herself and her child to begin building healthy self-esteem, based on true and authentic self-appreciation.

For Mary Beth, this meant noticing her negative self-talk, challenging its irrational, perfectionistic demands, and replacing the critical inner voice with soothing, self-accepting thoughts, ideas, and phrases.

By putting her internal house in order, she empowered herself to begin teaching Jonathan to soothe, support, and accept himself as well. This time, however, her guidance was useful because, at last, it was coming from a place of true authority.

Identify Your Ideal Child

Floating somewhere in every parent's mind, there is, or once was, an image of the ideal child we were going to have one day. These are the babies who never cry, the students who get straight to their homework after school, the teens who think their parents are cool. Ideal children all grow up to be highly successful, happy individuals, and they marry perfect people, too, of course, providing us with perfect sons- and daughters-in-law, and perfectly adorable grandchildren. . . .

Take a few minutes to relax and explore your particular, individual notion of your ideal fantasy child. Imagine the child at the same age as your real child. How would the fantasy child be different from the real child? Let your mind perceive the way the fantasy child would choose to dress, study, play, and interact with you. Think about your fantasy child at other ages. How would he or she meet your expectations?

Bringing the fantasy child forward into consciousness is useful for two reasons. For one, the qualities we give to our

Reactive Parenting

- I never got the toys I wanted—I load you up with material goods.
- I need to feel in control of myself—I pick on you.
- I feel inadequate inside—I seek your approval.
- I was a goody-goody in school—unconsciously I don't mind if you act out.
- I'm not living up to my potential—I have a high picture of you.
- I have trouble relating to the opposite sex—I obsessively pay attention to you.
- I'm very sensitive—I give you power to hurt my feelings.
- I feel anxious—you have a tantrum.
- I was helpless as a child—so I overdo for you.
- I didn't get enough as a child—I give you too much.
- My mother always told me to be careful—I don't let you ride public transportation.
- I always heard no—I have trouble saying no.
- I never heard no—I have trouble telling you no.

ideal child provide us a lot of information *about ourselves.* The fantasy child represents what we aspire to in an unseen corner of our mind. All its talents, qualities, and skills are reflections of *our* inner being, of course, because we are *solely and completely* the creators of the fantasy.

Second, when we clearly separate ourselves, our ideal fantasy child, and our real child, it releases an unconscious burden on our real child. That's because the unconscious notion of a perfect or ideal child can interfere with the vital, all-embracing acceptance of our real—and imperfect—child.

Enjoy your fantasy child *as a piece of yourself.* Use the information you get from thinking about it to help you identify what you want for yourself. But, say good-bye—forever—to this imaginary child as a competitor of your real child.

Who Else Supports Your Empowerment?

Nobody ever overcomes anything without the guidance, inspiration, or assistance of others. As social creatures, humans can inspire and sustain each other, or we can discourage, depress, and bring one another down.

After we take the time to become aware of our primary needs, and start organizing our lives around them, the next most important step to self-empowerment is assessing our social environment.

Think about the cast of characters in your life. Are they critical or supportive of your authentic self? Who understands you, or at least tries to understand?

Conversely, is there someone who is draining your energy, robbing your vitality, or causing you heartache? What can you do to make that relationship better? What would it be like if you calmly stood up to that person? If that's not possible right now, how can you avoid the person in whose presence you feel uncomfortable or weak?

You can explore your social environment by drawing a small circle in the center of a piece of paper to represent yourself. Put the names of the others in your life on the paper all around you, asking yourself, on a gut level, "Who supports and accepts me? Who approves of me? Who is positive in my life?"

Notice who is closest to you on the map and the kind of energy they inspire in you. If you believe that someone close to you, such as a mate, is not providing you with positive energy, or is actually bringing you down, you're going to have to assert yourself and make changes in the relationship.

You may have to sit down with your mate and ask: How can we support each other better? That's an empowering question.

Think about other people on the periphery of your life, too. Is there someone you would benefit from knowing better?

We each have the right to choose to be close to positive people, and to create positive relationships with others. We also have the right to respectfully stand up to, or avoid, people we find negative.

First Things First: Designing Your Moments for Enjoyment

Empowering yourself involves looking at every aspect of your day, so that your time is organized around what you find pleasing, satisfying, and worthwhile. As we've seen, paying this kind of close personal attention to yourself isn't really selfish, it's your right—and it's smart. When you focus on making your life as pleasurable, worthwhile, and satisfying as it can be, you empower yourself to help your A.D.D./A.D.H.D. loved one to reshape his or her core.

Most households with A.D.D./A.D.H.D.-identified children have better and worse times of the day. Your most vulnerable time is a good place to start empowering yourself and transforming the negative effects of the disorder.

What Gives You Pleasure?

Exploring the events and activities that you associate with pleasure is highly empowering. To start off your exploration, write a list of ten or more times in your life that you remember experiencing intense feelings of pleasure. What made these times so pleasurable? What were you doing? What did you think about yourself?

Make another list of things that give you pleasure, focusing on the accessible "everyday" pleasures. What do you do for fun? What do you look forward to? How can you add more pleasure to your life today, and tomorrow?

Sarah

At Sarah and Lenny's house, the morning routine had become a recurring nightmare. Seven-year-old, A.D.D.-identified Suzy seemed to be at her foggiest and most negative in the morning. The little girl hated to get out of bed. She totally tuned out the alarm clock, her parents' urgings, even the vacuum cleaner that her desperate parents once turned on in her room.

As Lenny showered for work, Sarah tried to rouse Suzy from bed. Every morning, Sarah tried to be a sweet and pleasant mom, but her feelings would soon be spoiled by Suzy's stubborn refusal to rise. Sarah would struggle to control her mounting anger as her daughter slept, pretended to sleep, or refused to get up. Sarah's patience would wear thin, and her morning communications would turn from pleasant to cajoling, to desperate begging, followed by threats, insults, and out-and-out yelling.

Sarah hated the daily haranguing and bad feelings this behavior stirred up in her. But when she was in the grip of Suzy's negative symptomatic state, she naturally felt as if she were being driven crazy.

By the time Suzy was dressed and ready to leave the house, Sarah was worn out. Driving her daughter to school, she'd grip the steering wheel with rigid fingers white with tension.

In order for the situation to transform, three things had to be done. First, Sarah had to really want it to change. Second, she had to stand back and take a hard look at the negative pattern. Third, she had to empower herself to take new and different actions to create new and different mornings.

In other words, Sarah had to take the time to rethink and redesign the start of her day. Until her morning routine was based on her own personal needs and desires, there could be no movement in Suzy's negative symptoms.

By actively deciding to approach her mornings by putting herself first, Sarah began the process of self-empowerment. She started by using her imagination to focus on what a satisfying, pleasant morning might be like for her. Simply closing her eyes for a few moments and asking herself what she needed in the morning yielded valuable clues and insight into her true inner needs.

Sarah realized that she needed a routine that would set the new day off on a positive note. That meant experiencing something pleasant, as well as getting organized for the day ahead. At night, she planned and became conscious of the next day. She learned to "see" what she wanted to happen before she showed up on the scene. Not only did she plan for how she would meet her responsibilities, but she also tuned in to herself, thinking about ways to add pleasure to her day.

Redesigning her mornings led to changes in Sarah's behavior, too. She decided to set the alarm earlier, but to linger in bed as she imagined the day ahead proceeding smoothly. She got up a little earlier in order to create more time for self-care, and even some self-indulgence.

As she searched for ways to enjoy the mornings, ideas came to her. She'd stretch her body to sensual music and indulge her love of aromatic oils. She'd cuddle with Lenny and, after rising, greet her image in the mirror with self-accepting, encouraging thoughts. Despite their high cost, she indulged her taste for fresh raspberries and other healthy treats.

Taking a hard look at the bad old routine, Sarah noticed that she had gotten into the habit of dreading the mornings. Upon waking, she'd been concentrating on Suzy and anticipating the negativity she'd come to expect from her. She realized she'd been spending almost an hour a day standing at Suzy's bedside, pleading with her to rise.

Another aspect of the bad old routine was Lenny's avoidance of responsibility for his daughter, and Sarah's underlying resentment toward him because of it. This resentment naturally affected their marriage in a small but negative way. Sarah approached Lenny for his help with Suzy in the morning. At first, he argued that he had to leave the house too early to help her, but Sarah persisted, in a friendly way, asking for his ideas and support. Finally, she gained his cooperation.

They decided that Sarah would rise first, to enjoy some time alone, and that Lenny would give Suzy her first wake-up call before he got himself ready for work.

Together, when Suzy was calm, they informed her that a new system was going into effect for the mornings, and they asked Suzy for her input in planning it. They stressed Suzy's ability to master the situation and created a simple point system which would record her cooperation and lead to small rewards. If Suzy didn't cooperate, a point system for consequences would be laid in the following week.

Through refiguring the family routine, Suzy's negative pattern was interrupted, and her A.D.D. symptoms could no longer control the family. Each day, her father woke her early, reminding her that she had to be up in a certain amount of time when Sarah would call. He set a ticking timer in her room to help her.

Sarah helped Suzy organize at bedtime what she would need for the coming day, giving her the freedom to select her own clothes (even though Sarah thought her daughter's choices strange at times). When Sarah delivered the final wake-up call, Suzy would have to get on her feet to get the good point. Since standing at Suzy's bedside had never worked, Sarah deliberately stayed out of her room in the morning, calling from the doorway.

As Suzy dressed, Sarah used the time to munch fresh berries and watch the birds out the window. To her surprise,

Suzy seemed proud of her ability to master the morning routine on her own.

This family designed, planned for, and practiced having better mornings—and they got them! Driving Suzy to school became an enjoyable time for both mother and daughter.

Sarah's putting herself first had resulted in transforming the nightmarish mornings into pleasurable times to enjoy herself and her daughter.

Empowering Affirmations

Affirmations are statements that we choose to believe and express. Through repetition, the thought being affirmed begins to take root in our minds and shape our experience.

Affirmations do not work if they sound impossible or untrue, however. Similarly, their power is undercut if they are said in a lackluster, unenthusiastic manner.

To make an affirmation powerful, state it or think it *with enthusiasm*, and *repeat it again and again* whenever you need to touch base with the truth it asserts. Many people find that stating affirmations in the morning, in a mirror, is a good way to start the day.

For example:

"I am alive, alert, and ready to live with pleasure."

"I handle challenges with strength and ease."

"There is a solution for every problem, and I will find it."

"I choose to be strong and calm."

"I am in charge of my life."

"I am a good person. My child is a good person. We are all good people here."

Teaching Empowerment

Once you get in the habit of searching out your true inner needs and organizing your day around your personal pleasure and fulfillment, you'll soon be an expert, helping others to do the same.

Your personal charisma and popularity will increase as well. People are attracted to those who are in the right relationship to themselves, living out of their authentic centers.

Empowered people are confident, not because of their money or looks, but rather because they have faith in their ability to know, accept, and love themselves. They live in the center of their own experience and take care of themselves in matters large and small. They also tend to be "down to earth," grounded, embodied, and secure.

They have a secure sense of boundaries with other people, intuitively knowing with whom to open up and with whom to act reserved. They can empathize with others but do not get enmeshed in their problems. They can be close to others without losing themselves or their sense of purpose. *They are comfortable seeking their own best interests, and they encourage others to do the same.*

As parents, empowered people become inspired leaders who guide their children into the realm of self-discovery. By setting their priorities on the positive, they teach their children, *by their living example*, to focus on what is truly important, and to align their impulses with their true intentions.

6

Sensory Integration

The path to better communication begins with learning about contact. You have eyes, ears, feelings, speech, thought, movement, and actions through which you make contact with yourself and others. Too often, people ignore the essence of this process.

Virginia Satir

Where the Body and Mind Connect: Senses

So intricate are the neural passageways of the central nervous system, where living chemicals spark and leap with every experience and emotion, that even advanced neuroscientists can be like grade-school students. This mechanical mirror of our minds is hidden from view, and owing to the thick cover of the skull its workings have been difficult to study even in our age.

The task of the nervous system is well known, of course: it is the part of us that collects and connects information from eyes, ears, nose, skin, heart, and guts—identifying, sorting, and drawing conclusions as it goes.

In our brain, thoughts, dreams, wishes, ideas, and fantasies all mingle, colliding and cavorting with feelings, from

161

the most terrible to the most sublime and tenderest. Sensations enter and need to be processed, and messages have to be carried from one part of us to another.

The messages we receive through our senses literally help us "make sense" of our world. When we experience problems or blocks in the way we process the incoming information, our lives will be affected in countless ways. For A.D.D./ A.D.H.D. people, unfortunately, these problems tend to prevail.

Sensory Integration

If you spend time around A.D.D./A.D.H.D. people, you have probably heard statements like the ones that follow. In fact, chances are good that you've made such statements yourself!

As you look over this list of complaints this time, however, consider the implications they carry in regard to the *sensory* workings of the person carrying A.D.D./A.D.H.D. symptoms:

"I tell him something, and it's like he doesn't even hear me."

"He can't sit still. Every little interruption and he's out of his chair."

"She's lazy! She just doesn't want to get up and help out!"

"He can't find his notebook even when it's right in front of his eyes!"

"He's so clumsy. He constantly knocks into things."

"If you tap him on the shoulder, he practically jumps out of his skin."

Every one of these statements describes more than just the state of frustration on the speaker's part; each statement also points to a concrete problem with how A.D.D./A.D.H.D. people use, or misuse, their sensory apparatus.

Sensory integration refers to the way senses are used to process life's experiences. Countless bits of sensory information enter our brains at every moment, flowing like streams into a lake. They come not only from our eyes, ears, and nose, but from every part of our body.

In our exploration of the sensory aspects of the A.D.D./A.D.H.D. experience, it's important to remember that no one has perfect or total sensory integration. Forgetting that my eyeglasses are on the top of my head, bumping into the occasional wall, getting ice cream on my chin are all perfectly normal occurrences. Nevertheless, they all indicate glitches in sensory integration.

With A.D.D./A.D.H.D. children and adults, the problem is that there are too many glitches happening too often. Information coming in or going out via the senses seems to get lost or misplaced along the way with alarming regularity. This misplacement limits the ability of A.D.D./A.D.H.D. people to perceive what is expected and make appropriate responses.

Only when the senses work together can the person take in the world with at least a fair degree of accuracy. When the information coming in from the senses is split off or fragmented, the individual involved cannot perceive or receive accurately. By focusing on the lack of ability of the A.D.D./A.D.H.D.-diagnosed person to properly integrate what's coming in or going out through the senses, we can pick up important clues about what conditions are needed to put him or her back on the road to healthy development.

Medical and school personnel who have not been trained in this area often overlook problems with sensory integration. Because the brain is hidden from view, sensory integration has not been easily explored in the laboratory, and many details about the physical side of sensory integration remain hidden and unknown.

Fortunately, through years of patient study over a period of decades, Dr. Jean Ayres of the University of Southern California has managed to shed light on this subject, which is so near to our experience yet so far from our understanding. (See Bibliography for more information.)

Dr. Ayres has found ways to map potential problem areas in sensory integration, which can then be corrected by assigning specific play tasks. When children are given the proper play tasks, stimulation, and activities to help them integrate their senses, their functioning in the world grows more appropriate and effective. In sensory terms, they are better able to be in touch, see clearly, and accurately receive and perceive the world around them.

Sensory integration is an area that every parent, teacher, or doctor of an A.D.D./A.D.H.D.-identified child needs to explore, for in the use of the senses we find important clues about what is needed to overcome A.D.D./A.D.H.D.

If we think of senses as food for the brain, then sensory integration would be the digestion process. We cannot get nourishment from food that is undigested, just as we cannot be in harmony with the world if we are not organizing sensory input in a way that is useful.

The A.D.D./A.D.H.D.-identified child who seems not to hear us, or is unable to locate something well within his or her view, is not being petulant or uncooperative. On the contrary, the child is giving us a vivid picture of someone who has a problem with sensory integration.

The hyperactive child jumps all over the classroom not because that is what she wants to do, but rather because her ability to process stimuli is out of control. The excess activity is a compulsive reaction to senses she can neither turn off nor organize. When the child attains the ability to organize the input from the senses, the unorganized behavior will cease.

Sensory Integration in Action

Imagine for a moment that the brain is a superhighway in fine condition—smooth, well paved, and without potholes.

Despite the good condition of the highway, if there is too much traffic, bad weather, or too many speeding cars, there will surely be accidents.

This metaphor describes the condition of many A.D.D./A.D.H.D.-identified children. Their basic equipment, the brain, is in fine condition, but because of developmental gaps (or poor nutritional support), the sensory input coming into those healthy brains is poorly integrated and therefore causes problems.

A good example of what we're talking about is eight-year-old Jim. When Jim was working on the PSD root points exercise, a bell rang in the outer office. Immediately, he swiveled his head so that he could "see" the sound, an action that broke the concentration needed for the root points work.

Whenever Jim hears something, his response is to locate the sound with his eyes. Naturally, this extra effort to "hear" makes trouble for him. When he is in a classroom where sounds never fully cease, his head is swiveling, turning, and bobbing all over the place!

The Sense of Movement and a Space of One's Own

Traditionally, we are taught that human beings have five senses: sight, sound, taste, touch, and smell. In this five-sense world, our eyes, ears, nose, taste buds, and skin make up the physical apparatus that takes in and gives out sensory information and messages, helping us to navigate in our world.

Upon closer view, however, two other sensing systems affect how we function, both physically and mentally. They are the *vestibular system* and *proprioception*. Becoming familiar with them is useful in overcoming A.D.D./A.D.H.D. because they round out our perception of what it takes to be in touch and in tune with ourselves and the world.

The Sense of Movement: The Vestibular System

The *vestibular system* is the way in which the position and movement of our bodies send messages to the brain. An example of the vestibular system in action is when a sad person decides to smile. The very action of making a smile tends to lift the person's spirits, at least momentarily. The vestibular system also detects the pull of gravity and gives us a feeling for where we are in relation to the earth. We feel the calming effects of slow vestibular sensing when in a rocking chair; it's the excitement of vestibular stimulation that we experience on a roller-coaster ride.

To experience the power of the vestibular experience, try this exercise:

Cave your chest in, frown, and let your shoulders slump down, as if you were in a state of depression. When your body is in the sunken position, try thinking a happy or positive thought—one that is based on reality.

We predict that your positive thought, *no matter how "true,"* will not sit right with you. *It will not have the "feel" of truth.*

Next, straighten up your neck and shoulders and let your head gently rise from the crown. Form a pleasant expression on your face, and think the same happy thought. This time it will probably seem a lot more truthful.

The only difference, of course, is in the use of your body—make that "the use of your *vestibular system*."

The vestibular system is operating day and night, sending messages deep inside that have been garnered from the way we move and use our bodies. It is a unifying system, basic to everything we do, feel, and think, as it provides a framework for our other senses and experiences.

When people do not process vestibular information adequately, they appear awkward and uncoordinated. Their self-feedback is negative, based on a sense of "I'm not." Their body language may send out inaccurate messages about their true intentions and interests, creating a situation in which the person is constantly misunderstood.

Physical insecurity or awkwardness is a greater problem than it might first seem, because nonverbal communication carries much more impact than verbal. Studies indicate that up to 70% of communication comes from body position and nonverbal communication, 23% from vocal tone, and only 7% from words!

Imagine, for instance, that you are talking to a friend about a subject in which you are intensely interested, such as what you did on your vacation. As you speak, however, enthusiastically sharing your experience, you notice that your friend is yawning, fidgeting, and looking bored. If your friend were to tell you, "I'm very interested," would you believe it? Probably not.

Children (and adults) with vestibular difficulties often send out inappropriate responses and reactions, the kind that do not accurately communicate their true intentions.

Another important aspect of vestibular input is balance and bilateral coordination, the ability to use both sides of the body. When we speak of a human being as being well balanced, we usually are talking about a quality of the person's mental functioning, but it's important to remember that *the use of our bodies both responds to and creates our mental state.* The mind/body connection is a two-way street. Therefore, the way we form and use our body is both a symbolic *and real* representation of our mental state.

Being physically well balanced helps us to become mentally well balanced. Similarly, the ability to use both sides of the body is important for having the full use of ourselves in the world.

For children, this is much more important than for adults, because *the human system develops properly only when it is properly used.*

The Sense of Body Ownership: Proprioception

Proprioception is important to understanding sensory integration. It refers to the sensory information caused by the contraction and stretching of muscle, by bending, straightening, pulling, and compression of the joints between bones.

The term comes from the Latin word *proprius* meaning "one's own." Our bodies receive sensations not only during movement (vestibular sensing) but also when we are standing or sitting still. Our muscles and joints send an ongoing stream of information to the brain to tell us about our position. *Proprioception is the sense of body ownership, or self-possession on a body level.*

Proprioception travels up the spinal cord to the brain stem and cerebellum, and some of it reaches the cerebral hemisphere. Most proprioceptive input is processed in parts of the brain with no conscious awareness, so we rarely notice the sensations of our muscles unless we deliberately pay attention to them. Nevertheless, we unconsciously rely on this important sense every day of our lives.

Proprioception helps us move. Without knowing the position of our hands, for instance, we could not button a button or turn on a faucet. Without sensing the position of our legs, we could not ride a bike or get out of a car.

The problem for children with poor proprioceptive ability is that they tend to rely on visual information even about their own bodies. They tend to have their eyes all over themselves, especially when given new tasks. This misuse of the eyes draws valuable focus away from the outside world, and the person's body language unwittingly sends a message of disinterest. A child with proprioception problems will feel disconnected, uncomfortable, and alienated.

Proprioceptive ability is important for having a sense of body ownership and knowing where you are in space and time. *Only when a person has a good sense of his or her body and its form and boundaries as well as its internal workings can the body function as his or her home.* Then, and only then, the person is truly embodied and filled—as opposed to being disembodied, "up in the head," and empty inside.

In other words, only when we are aware of the form and shape our body is taking, and the movement that we are initiating, can we be fully conscious and aware—not frozen, stuck, or lost in space.

Helping Children Integrate Their Senses

Expert neuroscientists assert that approximately 3 to 5% of American children experience problems in sensory integration. Note that this estimation exactly matches the commonly projected percentage of children who show A.D.D./A.D.H.D. symptoms. We believe that this statistical coincidence is no accident, because many of the signs and signals of sensory integration problems are identical to the negative symptoms of A.D.D./A.D.H.D. Sensory integration problems go hand in hand with the disorder, and a shift toward better integration is a giant step toward moving beyond A.D.D./A.D.H.D.

So, how do we help our children (or ourselves) to better integrate their sensory experiences? The answer is like the outcome of a complicated plot in a work of fiction—surprising, but also obvious and inevitable. The answer is: we can't.

We cannot integrate someone else's senses; that work can be done only by the person him- or herself. You and I always suspected that Grandma was wasting her breath when she said, "Stand up straight," but now perhaps we understand *why* her best intentions never changed anyone's posture. Sensory input—including the sense of how we form, shape, and move our bodies—has to be processed *inside, by the individual.*

In the case of many A.D.D./A.D.H.D. children, this vital internal developmental task has been interrupted—by any number of factors, from oversolicitousness on the part of parents, to the lack of available places where children can run free. To argue with the difficulties the child is experiencing, bribe the child with a reward, or try to point the way with words is useless: *problems of sensory integration are deep and unconscious.* Only new and challenging physical experiences will help a child overcome these difficulties. Fortunately, the kinds of experiences that will be helpful can be readily introduced into any child's life, since they fall into the realm of natural, uninhibited physical activity.

Signs of Sensory Integration Problems in Children

Auditory

- Child turns to "look" at sounds
- Auditory wipeout—child hears but does not connect to what is heard
- Child is very quiet or excessively loud
- Child has speech difficulties

Visual

- Hesitancy at curbs or steps
- Fearfulness of getting lost
- Inability to notice differences in similar pictures
- Difficulty seeing a figure against a busy background
- Difficulty following a moving object

Olfactory

- Cannot tolerate scents as well as other people can
- Cannot concentrate in presence of certain odors
- Makes little distinction among various scents

Tactile

- Child is defensive about being touched in general
- Child dislikes being touched on the face, in particular
- Child reacts poorly to many fabrics
- Distress at hair washing
- Unusual needs for touching certain items, such as a security blanket, while avoiding skin contact with people

Vestibular

- Difficulty keeping head up while studying
- Left/right confusion
- Insecurity about heights, falling
- Avoids climbing
- Dislikes being upside down (as in somersaults)
- Avoids jumping from higher to lower surfaces

Proprioception

- Avoids pushing, pulling, carrying
- Appears confused, lost in space
- Poor muscle tone
- Tends to be clumsy
- Complains about minor injuries more than other children
- Child is inflexible; wants things his or her way
- Blames outside forces for personal difficulties: "The wall hit me." "The chair is wobbly." "The pencil is bad."

So, What Will Help?

If we cannot direct, reward, persuade, or manipulate our children into better sensory integration, how *can* we help? The answer lies in nature, which has already provided a means for children to learn to integrate their senses: the way is play.

No one can organize children's senses for them. They have to do it for themselves, but they can do so only through their "play."

Big-movement play helps the vestibular system: sliding down shoots head first, jumping off swings, crawling through tunnels, climbing trees, running barefoot (so that the feet are in contact with the earth), bike riding, pretending to be a horse or an elephant.

Puzzle play is for the hands; folk dancing for the feet and legs; kites for the eyes and for proprioception; musical play for auditory sensing.

Play that uses the whole body is best for integrating the vestibular and proprioceptive sensing systems—leaping, jumping, hopping, running—play that most children don't get enough of these days. Experiences in big-movement play help the child to connect what's happening inside and how it feels, both to the outside world and to the grounding sense of gravity. Whole-body play establishes balance and freedom in use of the body. Sensory problems will naturally be corrected in play—if the right kind of play is available.

Work is also useful for children with vestibular and proprioceptive difficulties. Pulling, carrying, and lifting all help children to experience themselves as self-activating and capable beings, which is essential for moving beyond A.D.D./A.D.H.D.

Helpful parents will see to it that sensory integration opportunities abound, and that children have ample time to explore their sensory world. Helpful parents will be tolerant of children's peculiar likes and dislikes and of the inordinate fears that come in the wake of sensory integration problems.

With plenty of stimulating whole-body and sensory play, the vast majority of children with sensory integration problems will naturally correct their internal problem. For older children, this play may take the form of horseback riding, sports, skating, swimming, rock climbing, wind sailing, mountain biking, and other challenging physical activities that force the senses to align and integrate.

Activities That Promote Sensory Integration

- Blowing bubbles, Ping-Ping balls across the floor
- Hanging by the arms
- Pushing, pulling, carrying objects
- Bringing the knees to the chest
- Crawling
- Ball playing, Frisbee throwing
- Curling up the body
- Swinging, sliding
- Chewing, crunching (increases alertness)
- Sucking (soothes) (For an older child, try pudding sucked through a straw)
- Choosing fabric preferences
- Chewing gum while dressing
- If sitting is necessary for a long time, using an air- or water-filled cushion

Yoga for Children

The word *yoga* means "unity of mind, body, and energy"—integration at its best. Yoga is a wonderful activity for the promotion of sensory integration, as long as it is offered in a spirit of fun. A short exposure is best; under a minute is enough to spark a child's interest the first time. You do not need to join a yoga class, though you may wish to eventually if your child requests one.

Children naturally relate to animals or other life forms, and they usually enjoy the challenge of yoga if the adults who present it are relaxed and casual. There is no place in yoga for rigidity of the body or the mind.

The following positions are easy to learn and offer excellent opportunities for sensory integration, particularly of the vestibular and proprioceptive systems. Developing physical balance and the ability to stay balanced for increasingly longer times is highly beneficial for persons with symptoms of A.D.D./A.D.H.D.

Parents can learn the positions first, which will arouse the children's natural curiosity. Use your imagination to colorfully describe the features and quality of whatever inspires a particular stance. Offering a challenge such as, "How long can you be a tree? Do you think you can stay like that for a slow count of three?" may prompt children to focus and attend.

Yoga offers children the chance to accomplish something for themselves; it has many subtle and lasting benefits for core development. These exercises were selected from an excellent book on this subject, *Yoga for Children*, by Mary Stewart and Kathy Philips (Simon and Schuster, 1992).

Mountain

This stance appears very simple, but it subtly brings the entire structure into alignment. Physically, it entails having the feet firmly on the ground as the head, neck, and shoulders lift gently, the head resting on top of the spine. As you take this position, describe a mountain that rises out of the earth, its peak in the clouds. Encourage your child to feel the power of the mountain in his or her body.

Tree

This stance is super for developing balance and grounding. Starting from the mountain stance, let out a slow breath and place your right foot on the inside of your left thigh. Keep your weight on the heel of your left foot and think about the roots of a tree going down into the earth.

Put your palms together in a praying position, and slowly raise them over your head, like tree branches. Keep this position by relaxing your shoulders. Lower your hands gently. Repeat on opposite side.

Warrior

Warrior attracts boys and helps help to integrate their aggressive feelings into their developing cores by promoting strength and power without violence.

To begin, take the mountain pose. Breathing out, lift both arms overhead, with hands outstretched and shoulders relaxed. Step forward on your right foot, keeping the weight on the heel. Gently bend the right leg as you reach upward and forward, transferring all your weight onto the right foot. Let your left leg rise. Straighten the right leg as you balance, arms forward and left leg out.

Hero

A hero is brave and strong, and unflappable in the face of danger. In the hero pose you kneel on a folded blanket, knees together and feet apart, with your upper body straight and tall. (Toes point backward.) Lower your bottom so that your sitting bones rest on the floor, between your ankles. Then, link your fingers together and stretch your arms over your head. With shoulders relaxed, breathe out and stretch high.

Rest

Yoga teaches that stillness and quiet are as important as movement and action. This rest position is an excellent antidote to stress and frenzy.

Lie flat on the floor on your back with your head straight. Bend your knees up, let out a slow breath, and feel yourself "melt" into the floor. Cross your arms over your chest, and breathe slowly.

Big Muscle Play at Home

We parents, especially parents of active boys, mustn't love our furniture more than our sons and daughters who legitimately *require* active play in order to develop properly. Finding creative ways to meet this need is vital. The great outdoors is a good place to start, of course.

Opening the door and saying, "Go play outside!" is a time-honored way to provide children the opportunity to develop and grow, but when children have to be indoors because of inclement weather or because of apartment living, parents have to be more tolerant and creative.

It's too bad that jumping on a mattress will ruin it, but if you are lucky enough to have an extra mattress and a basement, you've got a good opportunity to create a play environment that can withstand action. We know two young boys who invented a game called Slippy Slidey by taking turns pulling one another along a smooth floor on a large towel. This activity busily involved them as they tugged and giggled in play.

Learning tumbling, rolling up inside a blanket and trying to get around, and similar activities give children the active play they need even when indoors. Save the expensive furnishings for one room, or wait until your children are older to feather your nest in style!

Creating a Pleasant, Sensory Home Environment

Because the seen and unseen aspects of our sensory world affect our moods and behavior, creating a pleasant sensory environment is a natural way to boost vitality, uplift energy, and strengthen us in our struggle with A.D.D./A.D.H.D.

To understand this phenomenon, pretend for a moment that you are in an imaginary room. This room is painted in a color you hate. A fluorescent light buzzes overhead. Around the room, there's a TV blaring, a neglected dog barking, the phone ringing. The voices of people nearby are impatient and stressed. As you stand there, the aromas of chemical cleaning products and overcooked burgers waft through the air. Chances are you are now thinking, "Yuck."

Now take a moment to picture the opposite, a pleasant room with a calm, peaceful feeling, a room with delightful sensory features. Perhaps there's a small trickling fountain. Mirrors reflect light on the walls, and birds sing in a nearby bush. The scent of natural rose, lavender, or lemon fills the air, and sounds of beautiful music are in the background. Any human voices here are those of happy children or of grown-ups laughing or gently talking to one another.

In which environment will A.D.D./A.D.H.D. have the upper hand? Which, instead, sets the conditions for a human's inner core development? The answers are obvious, of course—elusively obvious.

Consider this example of the power of sensory perception:

Imagine that you've had a harried day, your shoulders are tight, your back is achy, and your mind is racing, thinking about all the unfilled holes and hassles of everyday living.

In this uncomfortable state, you arrive at a classical music concert where you're meeting a friend. Your mind is telling you that you don't even want to be there, but you promised.

The music begins, and you settle into your chair. Music you like fills the space and begins to resonate in your body. Your mind shifts away from its negative chatter, focusing on the music and joining your body to take it all the way in. Your energy lifts as the music goes through you, and you find yourself holding yourself in better alignment, easing the strain in your neck and back.

By the end of the concert, you feel relaxed, in tune with yourself. You walk out of the theater with shoulders straight but easy. Thanks to the quality sensory input, your mind is now quiet and poised to be positive.

The point of this anecdote is to remind you to be aware of the power that sensory perception has on the human energy system. In our noisy, busy world it's easy to forget that we are essentially sensitive creatures who need to monitor the quality of our sensory input.

As parents we need to assess the sensory environment of our homes. The background sound of TV may be subtly pulling our loved ones off center. Even when they are not in conscious awareness, commercials represent a kind of manipulation that is dangerous to core self-development.

To counteract sensory perceptions that you find unpleasant, take an active part in creating sensations that you prefer. For example, going through the day tuning in to music that calms or energizes makes sense for many people.

Benefits of Music

- Largo movements balance brain hemispheres (creating opportunity for better learning)
- Music stimulates the brain and the emotions
- Dancing in the house lets off steam, releases stress
- Singing releases pent-up emotion
- Lyrics promote empathy
- Music provides stimulation with or without others
- Harmony tunes the mind and body
- Music sets conditions that free instincts

Aromas That Soothe and Calm

In the United States, studies conducted at institutions as diverse and prestigious as Duke University and Sloan Kettering Cancer Center confirm the efficacy of aromas in changing behavior and mood.[1] The effect of aroma is real, because of the close connection of olfactory hypothlamus and amygdala glands and the brain. Aromatic molecules in the nasal cavity give off signals that are modified before traveling to the limbic system, the emotional switchboard of the brain. There they create impressions, revive memories, and stimulate emotions. Aromas also have an effect on brain wave patterns and can be used beneficially to stimulate calm or alertness as desired.[2]

Because the limbic system is directly connected to the parts of the brain that control heart rate, blood pressure, breathing, memory, stress levels, and hormone balance, scientists have learned that fragrance is one of the fastest ways to achieve physiological or psychological effects.

Researchers have found that certain essential oils have a tranquilizing effect, altering a person's brain waves and producing a sense of well-being. Even aromas too subtle to be consciously detected have statistically significant effects on central nervous system activity.

In Europe, mainstream medical authorities rely on scent as a helpful agent in a wide range of health issues, particularly stress-related ones. Hospitals in England, for instance, regularly use vaporized scents of lemon, lavender, and lemongrass to not only make patients more comfortable, but also to help combat the transmission of airborne infectious disease. English and French nursing staffs are trained to administer essential-oil massage to relieve pain and induce sleep.[3]

When the Duke researchers put a pleasant scent in the air of a New York City subway car, they observed a 40% drop in pushing, shoving, and other aggressive acts.[4]

Once again, we are in the realm of the elusive obvious. We all know that when people walk in the woods or go to the seashore, fragrance is an unseen but powerful part of their experience. Yet, until recently, few have consciously used fragrance as a kind of subliminal therapy, by adding pleasant aromas into the home and car environment. Let yourself experiment with scent. Offer an opportunity for your children to discover their preferences in scents, too, and you will be helping them develop their emerging core and stimulate the brain.

While research indicates that any scent benefits mood and behavior as long as the person likes it, the following scents have been scientifically documented to calm and soothe stress: lavender, rose, chamomile, vanilla, jasmine, orange, and lemon.

Warning: Do *not* use chemical substitutes, which may irritate nasal passages, stimulate allergies, or add to air pollution. Instead, get your scents from the garden, from the grocery store, or from essential oils at a health food store.

Using Aroma

- Have children choose the fragrance they prefer, and put a drop of oil on lightbulbs in their room, if they wish.
- Use a spray-bottle diffuser for favorite scents.
- Use potpourri.
- Apply oils directly to the skin, or add to the bath.
- Simmer orange peels or a handful of dried lavender flowers in an uncovered saucepan.
- Drink aromatic tea.

Tea Before Bed

Preparing a pot of noncaffeinated tea before bed offers people a way to smooth the transition from waking to resting time. As a family ritual, the nightly tea, especially as a background to family reading time, is calming and focuses the family's attention on settling down and enjoying themselves in peaceful, quiet way.

When children have a chance to select the particular flavor of tea they enjoy, help prepare it, and carry it to the bedroom or living room, they are participating in a beneficial ritual that brings the family together without jarring outside interference. Nightly tea is an excellent sensory experience that promotes the opportunity for the calm and quiet mind to emerge. Combine with reading time for added effect.

Soothing Sounds

At the Center, we have a small water fountain in the waiting room because we've found the sound of trickling water to be soothing and relaxing. To the best of our knowledge, there is no scientific study about the calming effects of trickling water, but experience has shown us the value of it, particularly for A.D.D./A.D.H.D.-identified children, who tend to be attracted to water in all its forms. One boy saved his money to purchase a small, two-inch pump at a garden store so that he could have a fountain of his own. The soothing fountain reflected a part of his identity that had the capacity to be both stimulating and calming. Creating and using the fountain was a positive and pleasant experience that helped him to define, support, and integrate his need for stimulation and calm on a core level of self.

Signs of Sensory Integration

You will know your child is moving toward sensory self-organization and integration when he or she:

- Can play at one thing in a constructive manner for a reasonable amount of time (Children are *not* self-organized if they start one thing and *almost immediately* go on to something else.)

- Responds the first time you call

- Is able to keep his or her body still for a soothing bedtime story

- Enjoys quiet, relaxed conversation daily

- Can maintain focus when reading a book with chapters and few pictures

- Is willing to try different tastes, and if unsuitable does not overreact to them

- Comfortably, naturally, and automatically makes relaxed eye contact

- (Previously tactilely defensive) is comfortable being touched, and occasionally initiates hugging

7

Adults with A.D.D./A.D.H.D.

Wisdom comes when hindsight turns into foresight.

Deborah Rozman, Ph.D.

Adults are becoming part of the A.D.D./A.D.H.D. epidemic in ever-growing numbers. These individuals are deeply pained by their difficulties in organizing and directing their lives. Often they watch their peers move along in life, forming stable relationships in love and work as they remain entrenched in unsuccessful behavior. Fortunately, positive change is always a possibility once the individual commits to the recovery process.

Lois

Lois can't decide what she wants to wear to her job interview. Five tops are scattered on the bed, with a ball of stockings next to them, and her heart is racing. She's going to be late if she doesn't hurry! But where is the other navy shoe? It's not in the closet where it's supposed to be!

Cursing under her breath, she feels her stomach knotting up as she flings shoes aside to try to find the navy one. If she weren't so screwed up. . . .

A quick peek in the mirror convinces her that what she really needs to do is wash her hair. But if she does that, she has to use hot rollers to look really good. And they take time to heat up.

Still, she better be on time to the interview. The rollers were in the linen closet, right in front, but they're not there now! Pushing towels aside, she clenches her teeth and thinks, I'm getting crazy!

What she really needs is a cup of coffee—a good cup, not the instant type. Why didn't she think of that earlier! But it won't take that long to brew. Just put on the water and get the coffee ready. She's got twenty-five minutes, and the place is no more than twenty minutes away. And she can drive fast and still get there.

Lois races to the kitchen to put the kettle on. Coffee won't take long, and it'll help her get herself together. All she has to do now is hop into the shower. Her hair isn't really dirty, but suddenly a fresh shampoo seems vital. She's got to look and feel her best, because she needs this job.

She'll just have to figure out a way to explain to them why the other jobs didn't work out. A lot of people change jobs. If they ask too much about that she'll just tell them about her enthusiasm and energy. She got the last four jobs, didn't she?

Where are the stupid rollers!?

The blue top looks good, but it really doesn't go with any of the skirts or pants. Oh, just put the water on, and then jump into the shower. Being a teeny bit late will never hurt. Is anyone really going to be upset if she's three or four minutes late? Ridiculous! Just forget the outfits on the bed, they don't work. There's another dress in the back of the closet that will be perfect. . . .

Most adults who are officially diagnosed or who self-identify with attention deficit disorder receive the diagnosis with a certain sense of relief. Lois certainly did. Her life was filled with feelings of anxiety, anger, and edgy, out-of-control impulsiveness. Most people are occasionally frustrated by organizational glitches and disharmony inside, but for Lois and other adult A.D.D. sufferers, the glitches never stop. Lois *lived in* a place of chaos, frazzled nerves, and a whirlwind of negative thoughts, with little relief.

Without her realizing it, her breathing was frequently shut down, which in turn cut her supply of oxygen. She was like the rabbit who runs into the middle of the road and freezes. Only when the lights of an oncoming vehicle were in her eyes could she mobilize herself to run to safety. A life of running is intolerable and ultimately depleting; no wonder Lois was on edge much of the time.

And on the heels of her chronic frustration came the feeling of chronic irritation, which in turn lowered her already low self-esteem. How could she understand herself as a person who could snap at others and blurt out nasty comments? She knew she was bright and resourceful, but she was always messing up! What else could it be but personal failure? Sad to say, on more days than not, Lois actually *hated* herself.

If you have been carrying the symptoms of A.D.D./A.D.H.D. as an adult, then you have been hurting and misunderstood for a very long time. The foggy moments, the angry outbursts, the many times you took the wrong turn on the road of your life—at last, there is an explanation for them.

When Lois's therapist helped her to see that she suffered the symptoms of A.D.H.D. Residual Type (adult A.D.H.D.), Lois cried, right there and then. Finally, there was a name for her hurt. Finally there was a name for the intolerable condition of her life, the lost jobs, the romances gone wrong, and the impulsive behavior. Maybe now, at long last, she could get the help she needed.

Attention deficit that's gone untreated has usually wreaked havoc in a person's life. Like a boa constrictor, adult A.D.D. chokes off whole areas of a person's life—areas that should be sources of pleasure, purpose, or joy. Under all the frantic effort, the adult A.D.D. sufferer is often stunned, his or her core self immobilized despite the show of energy on the outside.

But getting the diagnosis of adult A.D.D., and getting *help* can differ.

Lois's therapist referred her to a psychiatrist, who started her on a series of medications from Prozac to Ritalin, Valium, and back to Prozac. Each substance ultimately had toxic side effects that Lois didn't want to live with, from headaches to heart palpitations. She had even experienced the desparation of depending on some of the substances. Once, when she was unable to fill a prescription, she had an attack of panic. By the time she came for treatment, she was on the edge of helplessness. Her core self was neglected and undeveloped, and she had lost touch with her very essence. Lois was lost in time and space and needed help getting back to herself.

No outside substance could ultimately stand in for a disembodied, uncentered self. Making the realization that attention deficit disorder was behind her many symptoms brought some relief, but it took a psychostructural shift to move Lois out of the condition and into a positive life, free of A.D.D.

Jose

After reading a newspaper article about A.D.D., Jose realized that the article described his characteristics perfectly. Meeting him, I (Rita) was struck by his unformed physical structure for a man in his late twenties, and how it matched his emotional symptoms. His body was all over the place—misaligned. It was as if he had no real shape and consequently had trouble being authentic and present. When he talked, for instance, he made no eye contact; instead, his eyes would dart away uncomfortably. He seemed to be addressing the wall on the other side of the room.

His physical apparatus lacked self-definition, which, as in all cases of A.D.D., was both the symbolic and real condition of his adult selfhood. His shoulders were narrow and raised in a rigid manner. His chest was collapsed as if he had to hold himself together, and his head seemed weighty. I thought he wanted to lean back and let it flop on the sofa but was forcing himself to sit up.

He confided, "When I read about A.D.D., I said, 'Oh, boy, that's me.'"

Jose's wife, Joan, sat close to him on the couch, a nervous look on her face. She explained, "I want to pursue my own career, but I'm afraid that nothing will get done without me. I've had to put all my needs on the back burner just to keep him organized."

Joan was trying to wear a brave face, but it didn't take much to see the hurt—and the anger lurking behind it—in her eyes.

Looking ashamed, Jose agreed with what she said: "It's as if I can only see parts—not the whole. Like, I was hired to design and build a fountain for a wealthy client. But the first thing that happened was that I couldn't even get into my workshop because it was so cluttered up. But when I tried to clean it up, it was impossible. I wound up getting so mad I ran out of the studio and slammed the door. And I don't know how to make it better."

Joan added, "I went in there to clean it up for him, but I don't know where things go either. I can't take it."

Jose said, "It's like I'm living in an Alice in Wonderland world, with everything upside down and distorted. And the more I try to make it right, the bigger the hole I dig for myself. Then I just want to go away."

"It's hard to organize the outside when the inside is feeling incomplete or chaotic," I remarked. "I wonder if that's what's going on inside you?"

"Yeah," he answered, "it's like I'm lost, and I don't know where to go."

Jose's face relaxed, and I could tell he was feeling a little more understood. When I asked him about growing up, one of the first things he shared is how he would run away from home at an early age.

"When I was three, I decided to move to California," he said with a sad laugh.

That gave me a clue to how long Jose had been suppressing himself on a structural level. Three-year-olds can't look their parents in the eye and say something like, "Look, I know you are doing your best, but you're not really connecting with me, or contain-

ing me, or giving me the consistency I need, because you never got those things from your parents. So, I'm taking off. I'm heading out to California to find a family that really connects. I need a family where my true and authentic self can safely emerge and develop. See you after I grow up!"

Instead, children find other ways of going away. Some begin running into the false but useful identity of a "bad" kid, designed to push people away. Others get away by shrinking or squelching themselves. Jose's caved-in chest indicated that, under the surface of his life, he had organized himself around avoiding as many painful moments of communication or intimacy as he possibly could.

I asked him to come to the edge of the sofa, and to take a deep breath. A small smile flashed onto his face as he did so, and I could see the color reenter his cheeks. I handed him a biofeedback stress test card to hold. After sixty seconds it was black, indicating that his energy was being held very tightly inside. If the card had turned blue or green, it would indicate a more relaxed state of being.

Although Joan had said she was the one who was organized, I couldn't help wondering if she had fallen into the trap of organizing her life around Jose, making Jose's work more difficult by enabling his poor self-organization. If she were standing alone, she, too, might have difficult prioritizing and directing her life. Joan avoided facing these issues, but instead put her attention on Jose and his difficulties. When I shared these thoughts with her, a look of recognition came onto her face.

Spouses of adult A.D.D./A.D.H.D. adults often have similar A.D.D./A.D.H.D. characteristics lurking below the surface of awareness. Their sincere concern for their A.D.D./A.D.H.D. loved one sometimes includes hidden agendas or serves as a mask for their own feelings and needs around such issues as low self-esteem, their perceived inability to organize around their own priorities, and feelings of inadequacy. At the Center we work with both spouses in the treatment of adult

A.D.D. whenever possible, helping them to organize their energy around their own self-empowerment.

From what they told me, Joan and Jose were living in a basically codependent relationship, constantly seeking validation from each other. I assured Joan that if she turned away from Jose's difficulties and started with her own, doing what she thought was important for herself as an individual, she would be giving Jose an important opportunity—the opportunity to face his own problems and look for solutions. By setting herself up as a buffer between Jose and his difficulties with self-motivation and organization she was unwittingly contributing to the problem. Jose had become too dependent on her, I explained, and it wasn't good for either of them. The first step for Joan was to give herself a break from his problems.

Jose let out a sad sigh and shook his head, saying that he felt hopeless. It seemed to him that every time he tried to do what he needed to do for himself, it turned out badly, and overall he felt like a "loser." I told him that there was nothing wrong with *him*: the problems that were making him feel so alienated, confused, and ineffective were coming from his actions and what he had learned—and failed to learn—as a child. I asked Jose again to come to the edge of his seat and told him that he could be in the center of the process of self-change.

"Well, sure, but how?" he asked, looking hopeful and scared at the same time.

I explained that he could learn to ground his energy and tune in to himself in a supportive way that would allow him to perceive the outside world more clearly, and open himself up to more effective, appropriate behaviors. As Jose followed my instructions, doing the PSD Jet Knees exercise (discussed in Chapter 4), his face began to relax and lighten.

I asked him to notice his breathing and to allow it to begin in the Hara point. I invited Joan to give him some space and asked her to join in herself, so that she, too, could get a sense of what grounded energy feels like.

Gaining a Different Sense of Self

Making the connection to the body's PSD root points gives A.D.D./A.D.H.D. people an entirely different sense of themselves and their ability to organize their energy.

In Jose's case, performing the simple exercise using the Hara point was like the first pebble thrown into the water, but I am always amazed to see how effective it is.

When he completed the PSD Jet Knees, Jose asked if he could stand up. I was pleased at his request, because I knew the deeper breathing and root point awareness were starting to move him in a new direction. It was both meaningful and symbolic that he wanted to get up, shift his position, and stand on his own two feet.

"It's funny," he said with a smile. "I feel better now. Maybe I have been depending on Joan too much." This communication gave me a feeling for how difficult it must be for Jose to stand on his own in the daily course of living. His habitual body stance reflected a disempowered, foggy A.D.D. experience of not being fully present enough to meet his needs and accomplish the task at hand successfully. When the body is aligned and the person has kinesthetic awareness, the body automatically and naturally begins to move the person toward more effective functioning.

After standing for a moment, Jose sat back down, the smile vanishing from his face. "Jose," I asked gently, "what's going on in you right now?"

"I just want to lie down or get away," he replied. "Come to think of it, this is the same feeling I get when I have a project to do. It's like I just can't stay with it." His answer reminded me of the A.D.D. children who have difficulties sustaining themselves in school activities. They, too, wish to flee or withdraw. For Jose, however, this insight, connecting his present-moment feelings to his everyday work experience, was an important step to self-understanding.

I responded, "Knowing what the negative habit is will help you to stay alert for when it comes up again. When you know what the old pattern is, you can take charge of it, reshape yourself, and quickly get back to what you need in the moment."

I asked him to lower his center of gravity, breathing deeply and allowing his energy to connect more with his legs and feet. "Let your feet take a stand, like a tree," I suggested. "Imagine that you are sending deep roots down to the center of the earth."

As William Reich, Moshe Feldenkrais, Ida Rolf, and others have brilliantly pointed out,[1] "it is the body that speaks the truth of a person's experience and the impact of the childhood experience on the present moment." Jose had never before had the opportunity to focus on himself as a connected body–mind system, and consequently, he tended to perceive himself as a victim of life's circumstances. By participating in the simple exercises, he was having a direct experience of his power to reshape himself in a self-supportive, self-motivating way. Color came into his cheeks as his body realigned itself as his focus went to a new and higher level of consciousness.

Once we start to allow our energy to flow and come down to our feet and lower half, rooting ourselves, we begin to become aware of a firmer base from which we can then expand. I then asked Jose to take the next natural step, to open up his eyes and look outside the window at a real tree, and to drive his energy through his eyes, outside to the tree, and hold that two-point connection.

By taking a long view in this way, Jose was creating a more powerful perspective within and without. He was not merely sitting lost in himself, talking about the things he couldn't do. He was truly focused on something outside himself in a helpful, self-organizing way.

By this time, his whole body seemed to become younger and stronger. His face seemed more alive and hopeful. These real but symbolic actions were just the beginning of a process that Jose and Joan would go through, of course. As they both became more conscious of themselves and their inner lives, taking their own stands for themselves as individuals, each was able to be better organized and more effective. Their tiny shifts in attitude and perception over time made a large difference in the way these were able to take on the challenges of life and find new, self-sustaining positive behaviors.

From his self center, Jose was easily able to take charge of the workshop clutter and his business dealings, making firm, quick, and effective decisions about what was needed for better functioning.

After just a few practice sessions, as he integrated these ideas and actions into his everyday awareness, Jose found that his attention was going where it needed to go. He and Joan were taking their own stands, so to speak, and spending more and more time in the right relationship to themselves and each other.

Joan learned to take her frustration with Jose as a signal that something was off balance within herself so that she could create the proper priorities to fix it. Usually what we say we don't like in others is actually what we need to work on inside ourselves.

For example, Joan decided to stop involving herself with the condition of Jose's work space, instead choosing to turn her attention to the condition of her own job situation. Their relationship, now unimpeded by blurry boundaries, could rightfully flourish and grow.

Jose is typical of an adult A.D.D. individual. His inner life and space had never had a chance to fully develop. His lack of grounding and the inability to perceive himself as the center of his own experience interfered with his ability to advance in his work life or enjoy himself and his family.

Though he tried to mask it, his lack of maturity and inner definition played itself out in his daily life, keeping him stuck and unfocused. As soon as he gained awareness of his inner world, aligning himself to his own body and energy, his development could proceed naturally and positively. Jose did what any adult A.D.D./A.D.H.D. people can do: get out of their own way.

Creating a Lifestyle That Supports Your Core Self

The ideas presented in other sections of this book, particularly about growing up, apply as well to A.D.D./A.D.H.D.-diagnosed or -identified adults. Adults who carry the symptoms of attention deficit were once children who, in the natural course of everyday living, never learned how to live at the center of their experience.

As an adult, however, you'll find that your recovery will proceed quickly as you learn to adopt a patient stand with yourself, tuning in to your feelings and needs and sorting through them in order to unmask false concerns and get down to the bedrock of what you truly feel, think, and need. When we are willing and able to strip away our defenses and face our genuine concerns we will naturally be strengthening and supporting our inner core. A rise in self-acceptance, self-esteem, and reality testing will follow automatically. This process of honoring our inner life is the beginning of true self-love—the kind that makes us better people, better parents, and better partners. Energy that was previously spent blaming, defending, or obscuring is now freed so that we can take the actions necessary to move forward.

The tools you need for recovery are self-acceptance of your current state, a strong intention to discover and develop your core self, and the persistence to keep moment-to-moment self-awareness ongoing. The internal grounding and

194 Moving Beyond A.D.D./A.D.H.D.

centering process is deceptively simple. Your body will be a good indicator for you because scattered, disempowering energy shows up in the way one's body and head are held and shaped.

Being alert to your physical alignment will give you a way to both assess where you're at in the moment and, more important, shape yourself into better alignment and therefore more effectiveness in living.

Our language offers many clues to the importance of this concept. When people speak of feeling "down" or being in need of a "pick-me-up," they are really describing a powerful phenomenon of self-shaping—one that is available to us at all times.

Ask Yourself the Right Questions

The human mind will strive to answer any question put to it. So, asking the right questions of ourselves is vital if we are to get the right answers. If a person gets up in the morning, looks in the mirror, and asks, "What the hell is *wrong* with me?" you can be sure that over the next several hours an unseen part of the person's mind will be searching for the answer to the question. The likely answer will be negative and destructive to the person's self-esteem as a list of flaws and faults is quietly assembled in the recesses of the mind.

Consider the following suggestions as better kinds of questions to ask of yourself. Asking these questions, and ones like them, will point the deeper part of your mind in a more positive direction. They will help you to focus on your center in an empowering way. As your mind searches for answers, you will be tuning in to yourself and adding quality to your life.

How can I create a good day for myself?

What sounds like fun to me today?

How can I help myself right now?

What do I need for myself right now, and how can I get it?

What is my biggest priority today, and how can I accomplish it?

Who is in charge of my life?

What's good about me?

What are my talents and abilities, and how can I develop them?

Where do I want to put my attention today?

How can I take good care of myself today?

What do I want to learn?

Adult A.D.D. and Care of the Brain

The process of recovering from A.D.D./A.D.H.D. is basically the same for adults and children. Becoming a person who is calm, self-supportive on the inside, and focused in his or her actions is not an easy task but is surely possible. As an adult, you have some resources, power, and information available to you that some children don't.

The first step as always is starting with yourself by deciding to overcome the manifestations of A.D.D./A.D.H.D. in your life. That decisive step provides energy for the next steps: understanding and connecting with your attention deficit behaviors, and then disarming them one by one. The out-of-kilter dynamics of attention deficit disorder begin to lose power as soon as you begin to make the process of centering and grounding yourself a moment-to-moment priority. Centering and grounding are not the end of the process, however; they are the beginning of an A.D.D./A.D.H.D.-free life.

If you have tried medication for your symptoms, you have probably reached the same conclusion that many other A.D.D./A.D.H.D. sufferers reach: drugs do not promote lasting healing.

Many A.D.D. adults, like Lois in the earlier example, try one drug and then another before reaching that conclusion. As with children, adults who take psycho-pharmaceuticals face a potential side effect of lowered self-esteem because of their underlying thoughts and fears about being defective, needy, or beyond hope. (These same depressing attitudes occur in A.D.D./A.D.H.D. adults who self-medicate with drugs, alcohol, gambling, shopping, or food.)

No one is beyond hope, and when the authentic self is established within an A.D.D./A.D.H.D. adult (by moment-to-moment centering and grounding), in time, negative symptoms fall away like dead skin. The process of moving beyond A.D.D./A.D.H.D. is the process of growing yourself up, stopping the action to reach for your inner truth, tuning in to a higher consciousness, and honoring inner self. It's a natural process that you missed learning somewhere along the line. It's a process that was always available to you, but not always accessible, due to the confusion of A.D.D./A.D.H.D. symptoms.

Pathways to A.D.D./A.D.H.D.–Free Living

When people learn to habitually tune in to themselves, alert to their own needs in a self-supportive way, to live in the center of their authentic experience, and to ground their energy by consciously shaping the body into the chosen response to a given situation, they're well on their way to recovery from A.D.D./A.D.H.D.

This work happens internally and can be done only by the individual. People are self-motivating and self-initiating and can never be forced to grow.

Many avenues can streamline and speed the process of becoming whole and free of A.D.D./A.D.H.D. symptoms. While none of them will transform the condition on its own, they can dramatically boost the progress of someone who is already doing the work of centering and grounding on the inside. Remember, adults as well as children with A.D.D./A.D.H.D. symptoms require more, not less, brain stimulation.

Following are brief descriptions of some helpful options. Chapter 10 contains other useful suggestions for healing as well.

Traditional Psychotherapy

Therapy can be useful for gaining access to deeper levels of mind, gaining awareness of unproductive patterns, and motivating positive change. Forming a relationship with a knowledgeable professional guides you through the process.

In a large national study, 80% of the people who had entered into psychotherapy claimed positive results in achieving the goals they entered with and alleviating mental distress. Brain researchers have even proven that psychotherapy has the ability to change brain chemistry.

Breathing and Meditation

As the link between body and mind, breath is a powerful way to promote change. Persons who carry the symptoms of

Breathing

- Sustains life itself
- Links the body and mind, and can intervene in the activities of either level
- Integrates different levels of being into a functional whole
- Is a powerful tool for expanding self-awareness
- Is both intentional and reflexive

A.D.D./A.D.H.D. tend to breathe shallowly, habitually depriving their brains of vital oxygen. Our brains are only 2% of our body weight, but they require 25% of the oxygen taken in. Unfortunately, the brains of most A.D.D./A.D.H.D.-identified people are simply not getting the fuel they need. Shallow breathing, the kind that is most dramatically shown in "fight-or-flight" breathing pattern of the A.D.D. population, also interferes with the creation and enjoyment of relaxation and calm. (The "fight-or-flight" response is discussed in Chapter 8.)

A focused mind is a calm mind. A person who is living in a basically unconflicted, harmonious relationship with his or her intentions will naturally have fewer negative impulses to contend with. Breathing is the ever-present vehicle that can blow the A.D.D./A.D.H.D. condition out of the water, so to speak. One simply cannot have a deep, calm breathing pattern and still experience A.D.D./A.D.H.D. symptoms.

Moving from barely breathing, with the secure sense of self barely alive, to deep, full, relaxed breathing that reflects our connection to what is good and true in life *is* moving beyond A.D.D./A.D.H.D.

Breathing Doesn't Come Naturally

People mistakenly assume that if their bodies need more oxygen, they will naturally and automatically take in more air as necessary. The truth is that the body will instead adapt to a lesser amount of oxygen than it really needs for optimal functioning and maximum vitality! In other words, we "get used" to shallow breathing, up in the chest. Shallow breathing then feels natural to us, and we grow unaware of the deprivation we are causing ourselves.

Shallow breathers are like wealthy misers who make themselves live on far less than they are able to afford! For the A.D.D./A.D.H.D. adult, shallow breathing has usually become the status quo; they have gotten used to and feel comfortable with breathing that deprives them of the full use of their brains.

Breathing deeply from the belly is the answer to this problem. The secret of making breathing work for you is to really do it, time after time after time. I (Avery) have had a client say to me, "I don't have time to take care of myself." But we all have time to breathe. We all can afford the time to become conscious of our most vital, ongoing, energy mechanism!

Meditation

Meditation is a natural antidote for the impulsivity and focusing problems involved in A.D.D./A.D.H.D. Meditating promotes healing on all levels of being—physical, mental, and energy levels. Some insurance companies, such as Aetna, have begun endorsing meditation as a beneficial treatment for many health problems. There is nothing mystical about the process of meditation. It is simply a way to quiet the mind so that the meditator can experience a state of mental relaxation and calm.

How to Meditate
Any experience that quiets the mind and heightens sensory awareness can be called meditative. Sitting in a chair with your hands resting in your lap can allow you to simply focus on the process of breathing, noticing the rise and fall of each breath. As thoughts rise to the surface, let them go, like bubbles escaping from a glass of champagne, as you return your focus to each inhalation and expiration.

As with other worthwhile activities, it is useful to build your endurance for meditation by degrees. An adult with A.D.D. symptoms can begin by sitting for a full minute or two, just once a day. Gradually add time until you can tolerate 15 to 20 minutes of meditation.

Meditation can also take the form of concentrating on a thought, word, or object. In this case, the word or phrase becomes a mantra that is repeated over and over slowly during the meditation. Meditating by focusing on an object such as a plant, flower, or tree outside your window can be a very pleasant way to move toward A.D.D.-free living. (See the groking exercise on page 127.)

Hypnotherapy

Adults with A.D.D./A.D.H.D. may benefit from an occasional session with a hypnotherapist who can help set the inner conditions that will calm and steady the mind, and lead to more deliberate focus of attention and impulse control.

Hypnosis is nothing more—and nothing less—than a state of deep relaxation, the kind we all experience in the twilight moments between sleeping and waking. The hypnotic trance is essentially the same state as that of meditation, with one important difference: in hypnosis, the relaxed state is used not to empty the mind, but instead to fill it with helpful ideas, images, and attitudes.

In the safe, comfortable atmosphere provided by a hypnotherapist, a person can focus his or her mind on upcoming goals, seeding the unconscious on a deep level with positive messages tailored to the individual. The person experiencing hypnosis is always in full control during the session.

Biofeedback

Learning to tune in, center, and ground oneself can also be enhanced by biofeedback, which has had promising results against A.D.D./A.D.H.D. in clinical studies.

It's useful for the adult with A.D.D./A.D.H.D. to become familiar with the working of his or her brain waves, the electrical impulses that our brains produce all the time. Being sensitive to our brain waves provides a way to begin sensing ourselves at the most basic level.

Brain Waves Made Easy

Here is a short primer to begin your exploration.

Brain waves are like different instruments that make

music together. Like musical instruments, they can be "played" harmoniously or discordantly.

At any given moment, we are usually producing a variety of brain waves. For example, when we say someone is in the alpha state, we mean that the alpha electrical impulse is the primary, but not the sole, wave being produced.

Brain waves are not "good" or "bad," but certain ones are better suited to certain purposes than others.

The four basic brain wave patterns are *alpha, beta, theta, and delta.*

- *Alpha* is the wave associated with relaxation and creativity, when the mind is receptive and nonjudging. Alpha is imaginative and visual, a daydreaming state of mind.

- *Beta* is the wave of everyday calculation, the chattering voice in our heads, which computes and solves concrete problems.

  When beta gets out of control, as it often does for people with A.D.D./A.D.H.D. symptoms, it produces a stream of thoughts that rush by too fast for us to focus on any one, creating an overall feeling of panic or of being overwhelmed. Interestingly, large-muscle movement automatically regulates excessive beta activity. When one is worried, for instance, and experiencing too much beta, a good biofeedback session will correct the situation.

- *Theta* can be thought of as the subconscious state, the part of the mind that forms a layer between the conscious and unconscious. Theta holds forgotten memories that still affect us and contains our unexpressed creativity, deepest emotional pain, and inspiration.

  Active A.D.D./A.D.H.D. symptoms respond well to the taming of theta brain activity. This can be achieved by deep relaxation with a focus on pleasant sensations or images in meditation, hypnosis, or guided imagery.

- *Delta* brain waves are associated with the "sixth sense," the unconscious, instinctual part of the mind that contains gut feelings and hunches. Delta gives us the capacity for empathy with others as well.

Taming Theta with Meditation/Deep Relaxation

Imagine that you are lying on a bed, deeply relaxed. With eyes closed, you feel the pull of gravity on your body, as if you were a heavy bag of sand sinking into the mattress. Conversely, you may choose to imagine yourself as being slowly filled with healing energy, with light, or with clear, pure air.

As you lie there, focus on deepening your breathing, allowing yourself to experience the pleasant sensation of deep relaxation. Your awareness of the outer world is still there, but it goes in and out, as you tune in to a growing awareness of your inner world as a self-created universe.

In this relaxed state, your stresses and problems fade, and you are gently carried into a dreamy state of peace and calm. You may visualize or daydream in this state, or simply keep your focus on your internal body process, such as your rhythmic breathing or slowing pulse.

This meditative state is a strengthening and healing one for adult A.D.D./A.D.H.D. sufferers, allowing the mastery of theta and beta impulses during a state of alpha receptivity.

Music

When the right and left hemispheres of the brain are producing equal, balanced brain wave activity, it is called *syn-*

chrony, or *whole-brain thinking*. Whole-brain thinking entails a balance between the hemispheres that may have more to do with emotional balance than we are yet able to scientifically validate. It is known, however, that during the most lucid state of being, one in which people display a high degree of awareness and mental clarity, their brain waves are almost invariably symmetrical.

As an adult with A.D.D./A.D.H.D. symptoms you may want to consider adding activities to your life that promote better balance of the brain hemispheres. Doing so is certainly possible and might even be a lot of fun!

Playing music, for instance, is an activity that is certainly stimulating for anyone's brain, and it just might prove to be an effective therapy for the alleviation of adult A.D.D./A.D.H.D. symptoms. The very act of sustaining focus and the discipline of practice will provide a positive challenge that counters the symptoms of the disorder.

Brain researchers have discovered that brain wave synchrony occurs when people relax and listen to music that is strongly rhythmical but soothing. Perfect examples are the largo movements of baroque composers, including Vivaldi, Telemann, Handel, and Bach. The experience of listening has an even more soothing and stimulating effect when breathing is paced to the music.

If you do not respond to classical music, listen to any music that is strongly rhythmical yet soothing.

Poetry

Another experience that boosts communication between both sides of the brain is creating poetry. Poetry calls on both the verbal and nonverbal sides of our brain as we reach into our deepest parts to find the images and fantasies that match our authentic feelings and ideas. Writing poetry can be a powerful tool for self-expression, one that builds brain power as it eliminates the sense of isolation and fosters acceptance of our fundamental humanity.

If you have trouble getting started, try this exercise:

Imagine that you are in a beautiful large house, feeling safe enough to be open to any experience, a joyful one or even a sad one. You walk down the corridor of this special place until you come to a door that has your name written on it. You open the door and find yourself in a special room filled with objects that have special meaning for you. Describe what you see on paper, and it is likely you will have written a poem.

Light

Making sure that you get plenty of outdoor light, especially in winter, is another way to energize the biochemicals that may be associated with the development of A.D.D./A.D.H.D. Repeated studies point to the efficacy of natural light in alleviating mental distress. Light is thought to be connected to the production of dopamine and serotonin, two naturally occurring neurochemicals that work against the symptoms of A.D.D./A.D.H.D. Establishing the habit of a daily walk in natural light, even in winter, is cost-free therapy with only helpful, beneficial side effects.

The Challenge of Adult A.D.D.

Adults who wish to move beyond A.D.D./A.D.H.D. have many avenues and options open to them once they commit themselves fully and wholeheartedly to change. Learning to find, support, and develop one's true and authentic inner self is worth the time, effort, and persistence it takes.

When inner needs are acknowledged and met, negative responses are no longer necessary. At that point, any remaining impulsivity can be counted as vibrant spontaneity. When energy is grounded, and the person is aligned with his or her true inner intentions, then hyperactivity becomes energy and fuel for a whole and healthy life.

8

The Toxic Trio:
TV, Junk Food, Consumerism

Television viewing is a kind of wakeful dreaming. But it's a stranger's dream from far away, playing on the screen of your mind.

Jerry Mander

I (Avery) have been conducting an informal survey for several years. Whenever I go into a classroom, I ask the children to put up their hands if they watch TV before school, after school, or at night. Almost invariably, the hands of the A.D.D/A.D.H.D. kids shoot up first and stay up longest.

This informal research matches a large study of TV viewing at the Australian National University, which concluded that TV is a definite, and significant, contributor to hyperactivity. So profound is the connection, Australian researchers learned, that *in rural areas where TV was not available to children from infancy to adolescence, hyperactivity does not exist.*[1]

The mechanism by which TV creates hyperactivity is as follows:

As children sit still, viewing TV, their attention is captivated by exciting, speeded-up, flashing, and often violent or brutal images that enter the brain via the optic nerve. The effect of these images is the stimulation of the inborn "fight-or-flight" response.

In other words, the viewer's body, though still and unmoving, has been flooded with the stress-producing adrenaline and cortisol. Because the child's attention is fixed on the screen, however, he or she continues to sit, passively receiving the images. During this time, adrenaline and other biochemicals associated with "fight or flight" continue to be released, and *they will stay in the child's system for hours.*

The trouble begins when the TV gets shut off. The child now has a body full of biochemicals that make him want to fight or flee. And that is exactly what he does, more often than not. With his biochemical system juiced up, he may reach over and release some agression by hitting a sibling, or he may simply begin dashing around the room in a reckless display of unorganized frenzy.

"He's being hyper!" the adults cry in alarm as the out-of-control child crashes around the living room causing trouble.

"Put the TV back on!" someone suggests. "He's fine when he's watching. TV calms him down."

And so the cycle begins again.

The Flickering Light in Our Living Rooms

In the average American household the TV is on about forty-nine hours a week.[2] Children view TV almost as many hours a day as they attend school. And when you get right down to it, TV *is* a kind of school, in that the time spent taking in TV images is certainly time that is being used for learning. TV is a very powerful learning tool, in fact. The question is, *what are our children learning when they watch? And does this learning serve them?*

Of the more than four thousand studies that have been conducted on TV's effect on children, the large majority have connected indiscriminate viewing with increased aggressive behavior, lower academic performance, increased fear of crime, and *lowered attention spans.*

As a quick exercise, go to your TV at any hour of the day or night and flip it on to a commercial station. You will see amazing things—things you would never see if you were sitting out on your front porch watching the world go by. Count the number of times the images change in a well-produced, thirty-second TV commercial. You'll probably come up with about twenty images, maybe even more.

And very few of those images will represent anything *real.* Instead, they are a dazzling array of pictures and actions, with dramatic music underscoring. The music is there to drive the intent of the images further into your biological system and produce what marketers term "a buying mood."

It's so wonderful. You're on a plane; you're in Paris; someone is in pain, takes a pill, and smiles. You're up in a hot-air balloon overlooking the countryside; two hands are coming together for a shake; a gun is being held against someone's head; the family is gathered in the dining room; you're overlooking the sea while a man tells you how good plastic is; two girls are giggling about sex—such a vivid parade of human behaviors, longings, hopes, and fantasies! Who can resist?

Certainly not most of the adult population. And certainly not kids.

The Effect of TV on the Brain

Within just twenty minutes of someone's turning on the TV, two important processes take place in the human brain. One is that brain wave activity slips into the alpha state, the receptive state associated with hypnosis and meditation.

At the same time, the amount of activity in the cerebral cortex, the thinking, judging part of the brain, is significantly lowered. In other words, as we sit, passively viewing, we tend

Myths About TV

Myth

TV relaxes people.

Fact

People become more anxious after watching TV.[3]

Myth

Daytime drama is harmless entertainment.

Fact

Viewing daytime drama is associated with depression.[4]

to accept the images that stream into our minds through the optic nerve, without thinking critically about them.

Human eyes were designed to see in 3-D and to take in information by scanning the environment. TV interrupts this dynamic process, putting us in a state that social scientists call *attentional inertia*. The longer we view, the less discriminating we become.[5]

Sadly, the descriptions of viewers as "zonked out," or "zombies," the living dead, are close to the truth of what goes on with us biochemically when we watch too much TV.

Should I Throw the TV Out?

Whether or not to do away with TV is a tough question, because obviously, for all its potentially damaging effects, it can also be a wonderful resource and positive educational tool. Some programs—mostly on commercial-free stations— really do instruct, and even uplift.

It's not that TV as a technology is harmful for children. It's the speed, the violence, and the way our commercial businesses attempt to turn our children into consumers that's harmful.

On the other hand, my training as a therapist tells me that children have to be a part of the culture into which they are born. Unless you live in a community in which a significant number of parents are also willing to live without TV, getting rid of your set may be too radical an action, one that would leave your children feeling unconnected to their social world.

Sensible Viewing

For children as well as adults, TV viewing—like most other factors of living—is best done in a conscious state. *Know what you're viewing, and why.* Half the time, you may discover that when you think you want to watch TV, you actually want permission to relax and slow down. Your child may be turning to TV as an instant and easy answer to the question, "What should I do?"

As a parent of an A.D.D./A.D.H.D.-identified child, or an adult with A.D.D./A.D.H.D., begin by making an assessment of the role TV currently plays in your life. Are you turning your set on to view something in particular, or are you turning it on out of habit? If you find the latter is the case, try reflecting on alternative choices before automatically filling your space with TV. It might be pleasant to listen to the birds outside for a while. Or watch for a glorious sunset. Or think back to, or review photos of, a vacation you once had, and savor the memories. You may wish to send a note to an old friend, read a magazine, head to your workshop, or take out some art equipment. The point is that freeing yourself of the TV habit will not only free up time and energy for your personal development and enjoyment, but it will also provide your child with a positive model of how to free him- or herself, too.

In order to promote and develop conscious TV viewing in our children, we, the conscious adults in their lives, need to guide their viewing. We need to be on the lookout for our children's emerging, vulnerable cores in relationship to TV. Ask yourself: *Are the programs and commercials that my child watches strengthening or cheapening her inner core? Are violent images frightening or deadening her on a deep internal level that goes beyond words?* Common sense tells us that the younger the child, the more vigilant a parent has to be.

Shows and stations that repeatedly strip humanity of its dignity really have to go, because children cannot afford to have so many frightening or cheapened images of living in their brains. *What goes into our brains through our eyes affects us profoundly,* and it's our responsibility as parents to protect our young children, to teach them how to defend themselves against media manipulation.

Detox TV—Tips That Really Work

These tips are really hard won, because I have struggled with the issue of TV viewing for years. Once, I let my children view fairly freely and also sent them to a baby-sitter who had the TV on a lot. The negative effect that TV was having dawned on me when I realized that my son's nighttime fears were predominantly based on frightening images that he'd seen on TV. At that point, however, he was hooked and didn't want to stop watching.

Also, video games had come into existence, and there was trouble in our home over that. My other son was fixated with them and wanted to play for hours. I have tried *everything* to undo the negative results of too much TV and video game playing. It literally took years to come up with a system that really works for everyone in my family. So I'm thrilled to share it with you.

We recently learned of a remarkable piece of technology that makes excessive television viewing *impossible.* The "TV

No More Zombies!

1. Remind yourself that as the parent, you get to make the rules about TV. If you decide that there's no TV during school nights or on, say, Thursdays, so be it.
2. Monitor programs and/or watch them with your children.
3. Tape your children's favorite shows (ones of which you approve) without taping the commercials, and let children view them when you are busy.
4. Communicate that TV viewing is a privilege, not a right. Without lecturing, share your ideas about the dangers of too much viewing.
5. Have children turn the TV off when the show goes off, or at an agreed time—without a fuss. That's the responsibility that earns them the privilege of watching.
6. Don't let children control the remote until they are mature enough to handle that responsibility.
7. Important: If instituting new TV rules is difficult because your child is already hooked, be prepared to ride out the storm of the child's disapproval. This may take weeks or even months. Addicts don't give their substance up without a fight, so stick to your guns.
8. Check your remote to see if it has a button that says Lock. If so, call the cable company and get instructions for locking out offensive stations. (You can unlock and relock them easily.)
9. If all else fails, stand in front of the TV and perform the rap song on the following page. Rappin' parents stun kids, which helps shatter their resistance to new ideas!

Allowance" is a small device that connects to the television to monitor viewing time. To watch TV, a youngster must enter his or her personal identification number (PIN). If a child has a TV allowance of seven hours per week, for example, the television will automatically shut off after that amount is accumulated on the PIN. This device encourages sibling cooperation and time budgeting, and does not interfere with adult viewing. We highly recommend it. (To order the TV Allowance, call 800-231-4410.)

TV Rap

Do you really enjoy having your head in a box?
When you watch too much TV, instead of brains, you
   get rocks!
Mr. TV ain't exactly smart, 'cause he's got a dollar bill
   where he should have a heart!
Just take a look around, and you will see, what
   happens when a kid watches too much TV
Gets fat from no action, gets dull in his head
Can't rhyme, can't think, the kid is rinky dink!
'Cause instead of a brain, he's got a little tube
Does all his thinking for him, turns him into a rube
I call that kid a boob, a kinda couch potatah
Just like a veg'table, in the refrigeratah!
Don't let it be you! You got too much to do—
Too much on the ball, to let yourself fall
For that fake imitation of life that you see
The fake imitation they show on TV
See, the world needs all of you to be on a roll—
Your heart, your mind, your body, your soul
And you need the world, the real world you see
So let yourself live—turn off the TV!

If your children haven't already fled from the room during your performance, shoo them away with those venerable parental words, "Go play!"

Stop Video Game Madness

1. Tell your children—without lecturing—why video game playing has to be limited. Communicate that playing is a privilege, not a right.
2. Have other, more constructive or fun activities available.
3. Make playing contingent on getting permission to play.
4. Refuse to have offensive and/or gory games in your home.
5. Make kids pay for their own games and rentals.
6. Set time limits, and stick to them like superglue.
7. Put the games away in good weather.
8. When games are off-season, take them out as occasional treats when you need some grown-up time.

The Food Connection

That food and nourishment affect human functioning is a proven and indisputable fact. Vitamin and mineral deficiencies, for instance, can affect brain functioning and produce a variety of mood-altering symptoms, such as increased anxiety or depression.

It is noteworthy, for instance, that iron deficiency, one of the most common mineral deficiencies among U.S. children, is characterized by a "marked *loss of attentiveness, narrowed attention span,* and decreased persistence."[6]

It is well known, too, that certain substances can speed up or slow down physical systems. We all know that caffeine is a fairly powerful stimulant, for instance, but somehow it's easy to forget that fact when manufactured drinks containing caffeine are so commonly consumed around us. A study of 800 children in California found that students who regularly drank caffeinated soda pop were much more likely to be identified as hyperactive by their teachers than children who drank soda without caffeine.[7]

In another study that supports the veracity of a nutrition connection, the *American Journal of Clinical Nutrition* found that adolescents with symptoms of A.D.H.D. had a significantly lower concentration of key fatty acids in their blood than symptom-free controls. (Fatty acids can be found in flaxseed, sunflower, soy, and evening primrose oils, and in cold-water fish such as salmon, mackerel, and herring.)

In the United States, many conventional doctors who endorse drug therapy for the management of A.D.D./A.D.H.D. symptoms are unwilling to consider nutrition as a factor in the disorder (just as they once denied dietary factors in heart disease).

Once again, it seems the experts disagree, with some calling diet an operative factor, and others claiming there is no connection. Since there is no definitive answer from professionals, we are reminded once more to become our own experts by discovering what makes the most intuitive sense.

Food Allergies

Allergies or sensitivities to certain foods or substances do not just appear on the outside of the body in the form of skin rashes, or reddened eyes; they can also occur *inside* the body, affecting functioning in many ways. A 1992 joint study between German and British researchers reported in the *Lancet*, Britain's equivalent of the *Journal of the American Medical Association*, suggests that food intolerance or allergy *is* a significant contributor to hyperactivity.[8] This study has been supported by additional research in Canada and Australia, making food sensitivities an important issue to be investigated in relationship to A.D.D./A.D.H.D. in our opinion.

We have talked to parents who report a startling change in their children's behavior when certain foods were eliminated from their diets. One that stands out is the case of an out-of-control eight-year-old A.D.H.D. child. Both mother and father attested that when their son ate a corn-free diet, his disruptive behavior lessened dramatically. "I believe he was allergic to corn, because within a week of eliminating it, he went from being a monster to a happy little boy." Those changes were still in effect three years later, and the parents could often determine when their son had inadvertently been exposed to corn products by the negative change in his mood and behavior.

We've heard similar statements from parents whose children were sensitive to milk and dairy products. They report profound changes in their children's behavior when milk and milk products were totally removed from the diet.

Allergies or sensitivities often arise with the consumption of such commonly used food items as corn, wheat, and dairy products. Testing people with A.D.D./A.D.H.D. for reactions to these and other suspected substances is well worth the time and energy involved.

While endorsing diet changes is out of the scope of this book, we urge you to consider the possibility that nutritional factors may be at play in the A.D.D./A.D.H.D. of your loved one. Diet considerations, such as mineral and vitamin deficiencies, food sensitivities, and allergies, should be part of any A.D.D./A.D.H.D. diagnostic work-up.

Taking Charge

The detection of food allergies or food sensitivities is made by carefully monitoring food intake for a period of time, noting the intensity of the child's symptoms both with and without the suspected food in the diet.

If impulsivity, lack of attentiveness, and disorganization represent the three most virulent symptoms of A.D.D./A.D.H.D., for instance, the first step in detecting an allergy is constructing a simple grid chart, with those three symptoms written on the left, one under another, and thirty little boxes for each symptom on the right. The purpose of this chart is to rate the intensity of each symptom by marking it with a 1 to 10 rating each day that the child consumes the food, for at least ten days in a row.

The second step is totally eliminating the suspected substance from the diet for another ten days while continuing to rate the intensity of the symptoms.

The third step is reintroducing the food and continuing to note symptom intensity. This simple process will provide you with concrete evidence of the effect of the particular food on you or your child.

Test Your Nutrition

Our bodies provide many clues to potential nutritional deficiencies when we know what to look for. For example, heavy vertical ridges on the fingernails may be a sign of insufficient calcium intake. Bruising easily may signal a lack of Vitamin K and a need to boost the intake of dark green, leafy plants.

Dr. Cass Igram has written a *Self-Test Nutritional Guide* that can help you assess your nutritional status and make improvements, if necessary. We highly recommend this guide for adults and children with A.D.D./A.D.H.D. (See Bibliography for information.)

Dr. Feingold's Additive-Free Diet: Fact or Fiction?

Food additives comprise more than 4,000 substances that manufacturers put in processed food to improve taste, color, texture, or durability. In the 1970s, Dr. Benjamin Feingold studied 1,200 hyperactive children by putting them on an additive-free, whole-food diet.

The results of his experiment, presented to the American Medical Association in 1973, indicated that the behavior of nearly 50% of hyperactive children was significantly improved (according to reports from their parents and teachers) when their diet was additive-free.

Ever since Dr. Feingold made his findings public, the issue of additives and hyperactivity has been hotly debated within the medical community. Many major studies, including one that involved tens of thousands of New York City schoolchildren, have supported Feingold. The smaller, but well-publicized, studies that refute his theory have serious flaws.[9]

By moving in the direction of providing your A.D.D./A.D.H.D. child a diet composed of a variety of fresh fruits, vegetables, and whole grains with a minimum of additives, pesticides, and chemical processing, you will certainly be providing the commitment that children require for their long-term health and development.

Junk Food as an Indicator

The nourishment that we put into our bodies says a lot about how in touch we are with ourselves on a body-sensing level. Most people enjoy a little candy or junk food from time to time, of course, but people who deeply care about themselves tend to support their bodies by making healthful food choices a priority. People who are out of touch with their bodies, on the other hand, may eat—even stuff themselves—with highly processed, or artificial foods. Often, this is done unconsciously.

In that situation, an addictive piece of the personality seems to take control, and the person loses awareness of the consequences of eating certain foods. This dynamic of denial operates outside of the person's awareness.

Our habitual eating patterns and the condition of our bodies say a great deal about the condition of our psyches and whether we are spending most of our time centered and grounded in our mind–body space or are living up in our heads. If we have gotten out of shape or out of condition, it's a fairly good bet that we have work to do getting back in touch with ourselves, honoring ourselves on the deepest level, and tuning in to our body-sensing ability.

Remember that parents and teachers who are not fully in touch with, and attending to, their own authentic needs (healthy eating is a need we all have) will tend not to be fully in touch or fully present for their children. This, in turn, diminishes the caretaker's ability to guide children in the process of healthy core development.

The craving of junk food or resistance to healthy eating can be viewed as an indicator of a person's inner sense of him- or herself. Just as an adult with poor self-esteem may eat poorly, children, too, express their love or contempt of self by what they consume. For some children, the consumption of food with additives comes as a reaction to social pressures. These children eat to please their peers, indicating a weakened sense of self.

Children who have been hounded about healthy eating may consume junk food as a way of expressing defiance to an overbearing parent. Here, too, the secure sense of self is weak, as indicated by the person's willingness to take substances into his or her body in reaction to someone else.

To the extent that children have internalized food (and other) commercials, their sense of self can be said to be weakened as well. A.D.D./A.D.H.D. children are particularly at risk for this kind of internalization because of their self-esteem and core development difficulties.

Little Consumers

The rise of advertising in America is unprecedented in all of human history; we are exposed to more advertisements and commercials than any other people at any other time in the history of the human race. Our culture is virtually steeped in ads.

Reliable sources tell us that the average American child is exposed to many hundreds of ads each day, from undisguised commercials seen on television, to hidden endorsements in films, car radio ads, magazine ads, and even advertisements now commonly carried on sports equipment, shoes, and clothing.[10]

Children, being vulnerable and unformed, have little resistance against this onslaught of commercials and therefore are a prime target for advertisers hoping to gain control of a growing individual's product loyalties.

Consumerism is an often overlooked factor that has a dramatic relationship to the development of A.D.D./A.D.H.D. symptomology, particularly low self-esteem. Understanding the dynamic of consumerism, and the effect on core development, is another important step to moving beyond A.D.D./A.D.H.D.

Consumerism and Addiction: the Link

Consumerism is a kind of addiction in which people are encouraged to focus on the acquisition of more and more products that are designed for convenience or the enhancement of "self-image." Consumerism has become a way of life in the United States, the driving force of our economy, and its development can be linked to the rise in the number of cases of attention deficit disorder.

In the consumeristic mind-set, the ideal state of being is "being rich," and the ideal activity is shopping or other means of acquisition. The addictive aspects of consumerism include the desire, yearning, or perceived need for something *outside the self.* The implication for those who suffer from the symptoms of attention deficit disorder is that the internal discovery of the core self can be displaced and replaced with a process that seeks meaning and fulfillment externally in self-image. In other words, *natural core development, in which individuals get to know themselves better, develop skills, and learn to construct a fulfilling life for themselves, is interrupted by the drive to be perceived as acceptable to others.*

True to the meaning of the word *consume*, consumerism uses up people (and natural resources). And judging by the behavior of the extremely rich as well as the merely wealthy, it seems to be a fact of human nature that we seldom if ever have enough. The longing for new, better, and different goods, and the overriding drive to attain them, that has taken hold of many adults and children is an addiction that will never be satisfied.

Low Self-Esteem, By-Product of Consumerism

The connection between advertising and low self-esteem, a painful primary symptom of A.D.D./A.D.H.D., is almost palpable. Here's how it works: Since the goal of advertisers is to convince us to buy certain products whether we need them or not, psychological manipulation has become their stock in trade. This psychological manipulation, which market researchers actively study and put into practice, leads individuals to associate certain products with certain feeling states. Through this emotional association, products are then used to enhance a self-image, or bolster feelings of self-worth, providing the consumer with a temporary lift in mood.[11]

Consumers with low self-esteem are better customers than those with high self-esteem. People with healthy respect for themselves don't have to shop for that special designer outfit to enhance their feelings of self-love. If a woman is sure about her inner beauty, she probably won't spend hundreds of dollars on beauty aids. A man who is certain of his manhood might be content to drive a perfectly ordinary car.

People with low self-esteem, on the other hand, will buy products to get that boost or self-image enhancement in an attempt to (temporarily) feel better about themselves.

Since children are in the process of growing and finding their fit in society, they are especially vulnerable to ad manipulation. If every kid on the block has a certain toy, the child with low self-esteem will certainly want it. *It is in the interests of advertisers, then, to create low self-esteem.*

The subtle—and sometimes not so subtle—message offered to our vulnerable children then becomes: You are lacking something; without this product, you're an outsider. Or, you are a loser, but with this product you become an instant winner.

If you doubt the veracity of this argument, watch some ads and ask yourself, what is the underlying message about self-esteem? You will be viewing psychological manipulation in action—and it's a powerful force to contend with.

Protecting ourselves and our children from ads, by educating ourselves and our young, is both necessary and wise. No child, and certainly not an A.D.D./A.D.H.D. child, should be exposed to a constant stream of messages telling him or her that the answers to life's challenges are out there in the world of acquisition. *Removing an A.D.D./A.D.H.D. child from the commercial environment as often as possible is a powerful act of parental protection, because no child will ever find his core self-identity anyplace outside himself.*

If our children are to become true masters of themselves, they must learn to think for themselves, make for themselves, do for themselves, and most important, look for solutions where they can really and truly be found, *within themselves.*

Walk the Walk

A wise saying from the Native American tradition advises us that if we are going to talk the talk, we'd better walk the walk. Nothing applies more directly to our adult behavior as parents, teachers, caregivers, doctors, or therapists in relation to our use of TV, junk food, and consumer goods.

Talking the talk is mere lecturing; walking the walk truly empowers us—and, consequently, empowers our children, who learn *not by what we say, but rather by how we live.*

Walking the walk means cleaning up our own adult lifestyles so that junk food, junk TV, junk toys, and the unending parade of desires for more, better, and different things cease being a factor. The more we can clean up our lifestyle, making it literally more *whole*some, the less we, and our children, will feel fragmented.

It follows that the more we exercise our personal power and provide our A.D.D./A.D.H.D. children with positive role models, whose main focus is on tried-and-true values like character development, the stronger our children's characters will become.

When we as parents and as people live in harmony with our highest, truest, and deepest inner intentions, the rewards are high for ourselves and our children. *And the habits we put into effect in everyday living are the most powerful "ads" of all, for they represent our actual and true endorsement and promotion of a wholesome, healthy lifestyle—a lifestyle that encourages and supports the full emergence and development of a secure inner self.*

9

Antidotes

Above all, do no harm . . .

Hippocrates

No one wants to hurt. No one wants to stand passively by as their child or loved one struggles with life and appears to be losing. Looking for relief, we turn to antidotes in times of trouble. This chapter will provide an in-depth look at the remedy most commonly prescribed to control A.D.D./A.D.H.D. symptoms—methylphenidate, or Ritalin—and introduce other potential aids to recovery as well.

If Only . . .

Ritalin is *awesome*. What a relief! It's a substance that makes fretfulness, petulance, inattention, and childish defiance go away—and it does so almost instantaneously! With Ritalin, a child who was foggy, cranky, annoying, or otherwise distressed becomes calm, focused, and compliant. He no longer disrupts the classroom. Out of school, he behaves well, even when visiting relatives with crystal figurine collections. With Ritalin, children who are lost in the fog of inattention become sharper and able to focus on details.

No wonder 10 million American children line up for their doses of Ritalin every day. No wonder millions of other

223

parents wonder if they, too, should provide the drug for their children. After all, most doctors recommend Ritalin for children who show the symptoms of A.D.D. And so many doctors and parents couldn't possibly be mistaken . . . could they?

The Risks Versus the Benefits

When doctors talk about the benefits of Ritalin, they are on firm footing. Clinical tests have proven that with Ritalin, about 70% of children who carry the symptoms of attention deficit will become calmer and more focused—for the time that the substance is in their bodies, at least. No one, however, *not even the maker of the drug,* will tell you that the benefits alter A.D.D./A.D.H.D. symptoms in the long run.

If you are considering putting your child "on" Ritalin, or any other psychopharmaceutical, or if you have already taken that step, your actions are completely understandable. Your child needed help to function, and with Ritalin, you could get it in a hurry. Chances are you were feeling frustrated and helpless when you took your child in for a medical evaluation.

An A.D.D. or A.D.H.D. diagnosis does not appear out of the blue; it's been in the works for some time, coming at the end of a long chain of frustrating, miserable moments for parent and child. By the time parents seek professional help, emotions have usually been running high for some time. Parents who feel desperate naturally will reach for desperate solutions.

You may have first learned about Ritalin from someone who used it with success. And when you consulted with your personal physician, asking his or her opinion about the appropriateness of giving Ritalin to your child, your physician engaged you in a serious discussion before writing out the prescription, or offering to do so.

You were probably concerned about any possible side effects, and when you asked about them, your doctor took your concern seriously. He or she may have informed you that *all* drugs have side effects—and that the larger question is whether the benefits of the substance outweigh the risks.

Your doctor was doing his or her best, trying to ease your distress and help your child, by taking the approach that was taught in medical school, an approach to wellness called *allopathy.*

Allopathy, the standard medical practice of the United States, is a branch of medicine that seeks to correct physiological malfunctions and imbalances, and relieve patients' symptoms, by altering the internal body chemistry or structure. Prescribing a substance is the first line of action taken by most allopathic doctors (surgery is the second). In allopathic medicine, prescription drugs are the number-one symptom-relieving operatives.

By suggesting a prescription for a child, doctors are doing what they truly think best. They are able to recommend Ritalin with confidence because they know that the drug actually delivers the goods in the majority of cases. But what are the risks?

What Is Ritalin? And Why Does It Work?

Ritalin is a central nervous system (brain) stimulant, and a close relative of the amphetamine family, that goes by the scientific name of methylphenidate. Because of its amphetamine-like structure, the U.S. Drug Enforcement Agency (DEA) classifies Ritalin as a "highly addictive controlled substance," in the same category as cocaine, methadone, and methamphetamine, the street name of which is "speed."

In addition, the DEA has laid down strict regulations designed to keep Ritalin off the streets, where, as "Vitamin R," it has become an attractive product to drug users and dealers. The DSM, the document that has defined and standardized the diagnosis of A.D.D./A.D.H.D., reports that "controlled studies have shown that experienced users are unable to distinguish amphetamine (such as Ritalin) from cocaine."

Ritalin has been around since the 1940s and was once, at higher doses, a preferred "diet" pill. Hailed now as a major antidote for alleviating the symptoms of A.D.D./A.D.H.D., the drug has enjoyed a resurgence in use, becoming a common feature in many schools and homes. Like junior members of "Prozac nation," 6 million young Americans line up every day for their doses of Ritalin. The profit that this activity generates is in the hundreds of millions of dollars per year.

As for why Ritalin ameliorates the symptoms of A.D.D. in children, the bottom-line truth is that no one—not even the maker of the drug—fully understands why or how it works. One would not expect a calming effect to be produced by a central nervous system stimulant, for instance, but paradoxically, Ritalin calms children—*all* children, by the way, not just the ones diagnosed with A.D.D. or A.D.H.D.[1]

Many in the medical profession are concerned that American children are being overmedicated for problems that are essentially problems in living. This concern became alarm at one point in 1995 after a spate of sudden deaths of children who were taking a combination of Ritalin and Clonodine.[2]

Only in America

The widespread use of Ritalin and other psychopharmaceutical agents is largely an American phenomenon. American children are fifteen times more likely to be given drugs for their behavior difficulties than their European counterparts, for instance. In Europe, the idea of medicating children with psychoactive substances, except in cases of life-threatening emergency, is generally viewed as dangerous and abhorrent.

Out of concern, the International Narcotics Control Board has issued a substantive report about the "overuse" of methylphenidate as a "quick solution" for troublesome behavior in children and warns that the drug "could pose dangers to the children's well-being over time."[3]

Dr. Arthur Caplan, director of the Center for Bioethics at the University of Pennsylvania, has similarly expressed his concern about the explosion of A.D.D./A.D.H.D. diagnoses and the attendant drug prescriptions that both children and adults are being given. He noted: "The fact that a similar explosion is not taking place in other parts of the world is suspicious: why would only Americans be afflicted with this? And why are only Americans being treated? I think we need to step back and take another look."[4]

We agree. And we strongly believe that two key points need to be kept firmly in mind:

1. The feeling of perceived defect in the core of the self is the basis for all chronic emotional suffering, and

2. No substance will ever substitute for being attuned with one's own secure sense of self.

Side Effects—Common and Uncommon

When we speak of a substance's "side" effects, we are really referring to its *total* effect. All drugs have effects upon the body. Some of those effects are the ones we're looking for, and others—the side effects—are unsought and unwanted.

One of the most common side effects of Ritalin according to doctors, parents, and teachers, for instance, is the "rebound" effect. "Rebounding" refers to negative changes in mood, increased irritability, and behavior and attention problems when the drug wears off. Could this be connected to the drug's known addictive qualities? Think of a nicotine addict without cigarettes and you'll have an idea of what the rebound effect looks, feels, and acts like.

Another common side effect is weight loss. That's not surprising when you consider that Ritalin began as a diet pill—

it's well known that amphetamines suppress appetite. But let's take it a step further: what does the effect of weight loss mean for *growing children*? Research indicates that children taking Ritalin on a long-term basis (two to four years) experience a 2% loss in height compared with their peers.[5] Fortunately, children who have taken the drug for two years or less tend to make up that growth—but only *after the drug is discontinued.*

Difficulty sleeping and changes in heart rate, heart rhythm, and blood pressure are other effects of Ritalin. *To refer to them as "side" effects hardly seems accurate given that these effects are so common in amphetamine and amphetamine-like drugs.*

Whenever a drug is purchased in the United States, a printed insert is put in the package that describes the substance, how it works, and how it should be used. This insert, which is required by the Food and Drug Administration (FDA), contains the same information that your doctor is given in the authoritative *Physician's Desk Reference* (PDR).

If you are considering whether to give your child Ritalin, Cylert, Clonodine, or another medication to relieve the symptoms of attention deficit disorder, you need to make an informed choice. That means taking advantage of your right to know, by reading the fine print. Here is an excerpt of the fine print about Ritalin:

Ritalin

The mode of action in man is not completely understood, but Ritalin presumably activates the brain stem arousal system.

WARNING: Ritalin should not be used in children under 6 years, since safety and efficacy in this group has not been established. Sufficient data on safety and efficacy of long-term use are not yet available. Suppression of growth (i.e. height and weight gain) has been reported with the long-term use of this stimulant. Symptoms of visual disturbances have been encountered in rare cases. Blurring of vision has been reported.

ADVERSE REACTIONS: Nervousness and insomnia are the most common adverse reactions. Other reactions include skin rash, fever, headache, dyskinesia (involuntary movement), drowsiness, blood pressure and pulse changes, both up and down, tachycardia (rapid heart beat), angina, cardia arrhythmia (irregular heartbeat), abdominal pain, reduction of clotting platelets, and weight loss. There have been reports of Tourette's Syndrome.[6] Toxic psychosis has been reported. Although a definite causal relationship has not been established, the following have been reported in patients taking this drug: cerebral occlusion, leukopenia (loss of white blood cells) and/or anemia, depressed mood, scalp hair loss. Any of the adverse reactions listed above may occur.

CONTRAINDICATIONS (Authors' note: contraindication advises a doctor *not* to offer a particular medication when certain other factors are in operation.) Marked anxiety, tension, and *agitation* are contraindications to Ritalin *since the drug may aggravate these symptoms* (emphasis added).

Source: Food and Drug Administration

Strange but True

It's strange to think that a drug that is contraindicated in cases of *agitation* would be given to hyperactive children. The distinction between agitation and hyperactivity is surely a very fine one. Similarly, the side effect of insomnia alone would seem to preclude the effectiveness for the substance in children. Nevertheless, the world of A.D.D./A.D.H.D. is filled with contradictions and paradoxes like these.

Another report indicates that children taking Ritalin are prone to entering a state of perseveration. In mental health terms, *perseveration* is the condition of doggedly pursuing an action or activity despite the lack of productivity. This is the situation of someone who is "trying too hard" and trying the same way, over and over, with no satisfying results.

The Ritalin Cancer Risk for Children

In 1996, as we prepared the first edition of this book, we reported on the scientific studies linking Ritalin and similar drugs to increased liver cancer in mice. The quick response of the pharmaceutical proponents was, "Children are not mice." Representatives of the pharmaceutical establishment did what they often do when disturbing news arises. They called for more studies.

Now, as we are in the process of preparing the second edition of Moving Beyond ADD/ADHD, a new study has emerged. This time an important cancer risk factor was connected to Ritalin use in children.

Researchers at the University of Texas M. D. Anderson Cancer Center in Houston and the UT Medical Branch in Galveston were concerned that even though methylphenidate has been approved for human use for more than 50 years, there are surprisingly few studies on the potential of serious side effects, such as genetic mutation or cancer.

To learn more, they devised a study that recruited twelve youngsters who were newly diagnosed with Attention Deficit problems. They drew blood from these youngsters before treatment and then again, three months later.

The results were startling, and should concern us all: After being given the drug, each and every one of the Texas children had developed a kind of chromosomal damage that is known to be associated with increased risk for cancer.

Reading the Fine Print

Since the first edition of this book, other drugs that have been commonly prescribed for ADD/ADHD symptoms have been withdrawn from the market. Adderall has been banned in Canada since 2004, when it was implicated in 14 deaths, and the makers of Cylert, a drug that we had warned readers about in 1997, have announced that they will discontinue the drug after more disturbing reports of liver damage surfaced.

Anyone who carefully read the fine print on the package insert of these drugs could have learned of their potentially harmful side effects, yet amazingly, many people are willing to blow off that important information.

When we suggested reading the package insert about an ADD/ADHD drug, one father cavalierly tossed off our suggestion. "Oh, if you read the fine print on any drug, even over the counter stuff, you'd never take any of it."

True enough. But we seldom take over the counter drugs day after day as ADD/ADHD drugs are prescribed.

Can we really afford to stick our heads in the sand about the potential dangers of drugs that treat behavior? Do we really want to take such serious risks with our precious children?

The Most Insidious Side Effect

In our opinion, one of the worst and most common side effects of ADD drugs is not listed by the FDA. It's the subtle but serious negative effect on a child's self-identity. When children are given medication to help them correct their behavior, the unspoken conclusion that they draw is that there is something "wrong" with them, or that they have some kind of deep, internal deficiency or defect.

All children are vulnerable to the opinions of the adults who care for them. They hear the meaning beneath our words and feel our concerns and fears very keenly.

Perhaps you can remember back to the days of your childhood and recall how a grown-up's comments and opinions affected you. Many a budding musician has been

Too Close for Comfort

This chart compares the physiological effects of Ritalin
and cocaine as reported by researchers at Harvard Medical
School.

Methylphenidate (Ritalin)	Cocaine
Inhibits reabsorption of dopamine	Inhibits reabsorption of dopamine
Functions as a brain stimulant	Functions as a brain stimulant
Affects the corpus striatum	Affects the corpus striatum
Enters brain in four to six minutes	Enters brain in four to six minutes
Reaches peak level in four to ten minutes	Reaches peak level in two to eight minutes
Peak concentration lasts fifteen to twenty minutes	Peak concentration lasts two to four minutes
Half remains in brain for ninety minutes	Half remains in brain for twenty minutes

Note: When cocaine is administered orally, it remains in the
brain approximately as long as methylphenidate.

thwarted by an unkind comment when the child was practicing an instrument, for instance. Conversely, a small positive comment about something a child is doing can open the
door to a lifelong interest.

How, then, must it feel to a child to be taking medication to alleviate the symptoms of attention deficit disorder?
If you have a child, or know of a child, receiving medication, take a moment to try to imagine how that child must
feel about him- or herself.

How can we expect our children to understand a psychosocial disorder that the nation's leading scientists and researchers cannot fully comprehend? Imagine yourself overhearing talk about your "disorder" or "disability." Even if they attempted to mask it, wouldn't you pick up on your parents' concern?

What would it feel like to be labeled at school and at home? Perhaps you have come across a popular workbook for A.D.D./A.D.H.D. kids that tells you that the initials A.D.H.D. "could stand for Awesome, Determined, Happy, and Dazzling." Would you be reassured by this blatant attempt to mask the truth? Or would you feel that there is something radically wrong with you?

Putting yourself in the shoes of an A.D.D./A.D.H.D.-diagnosed child may not be comfortable, but the exercise in empathy will offer you understanding that is valuable and real. *No substance will ever substitute for a secure sense of self.*

Vitamin R

Vitamin R is the street name for Ritalin. It's the name that's used when the drug is peddled illegally to college students who want to study, or who "need" it to drive cross-country on very little sleep. The source of Vitamin R is prescriptions that have been hijacked. A younger sibling's tablets may be pilfered and sold on the playground, only to be crushed into powder suitable for snorting by adolescents.

Vitamin R is a drug that is growing in popularity, particularly with young people who want to achieve. Sadly, it's also a popular drug for parents who want their children to succeed.

I bumped into one mother who had come to an initial meeting at the Center but had decided not to pursue therapy for her child. "He's still on Ritalin," the mother said. "But what can I do? He's getting all *A*s!" This parent was operating under the mistaken belief that Ritalin increases academic achievement. Every clinical study done on this topic refutes that belief.

Cause for Concern

A study of "Cortical Atrophy in Young Adults," published in the professional journal *Psychiatric Research*, found that brain tissue shrinkage had occurred in *more than half* of twenty-four young adults who had been give medication as children. The 1986 study concluded that "cortical atrophy may be a long-term adverse effect of this (stimulant) treatment."[8]

As Dr. Peter Breggin points out, one study is merely suggestive, not conclusive. Is this a risk worth taking? We think not.

Stimulants have not yet been demonstrated to have long-term effects (on A.D.D./A.D.H.D.). . . . Clearly, medication is not sufficient treatment.

Dr. M. Dulcon, Textbook of Psychiatry, *American Psychiatric Press*

We seem to think that to name a disease is to understand it, to classify is to conquer it, and to suppress its symptoms with drugs is to cure it. How could we, the healing profession, be so utterly wrong?

Dr. Majid Ali, RDA: Rats, Drugs and Assumptions, *1995*

The most successful patients are those who live healthfully and avoid drugs until every other option has been explored (except in emergency situations). Drugs often mask symptoms while leaving the true cause of the problem to grow worse.

Meir Schneider, Self-Healing, *1989*

Ritalin as a Placebo

The idea of taking Ritalin to "gain control of one's impulses" has been found in several studies to be a potent placebo in and of itself. One California study found that boys who thought they were being given Ritalin (they actually received a harmless placebo) predicted that they would perform certain computer tasks more easily. Boys who had taken the placebo rated their experience as far more positive when they *thought* they had taken Ritalin. The placebo effect of believing one is taking a drug that will help one become more competent is very strong, but ultimately a trap.

In our experience, children taking Ritalin have one more reason to be looking for self-structure outside of themselves instead of inside where true empowerment takes place. As long as the power and organization are experienced as coming from outside the self, any change in behavior will be superficial and temporary.

Alternatives to Ritalin

The best alternative to Ritalin, and the only path to healing A.D.D./A.D.H.D., is the development of a secure sense of self deep within. This sense of self will naturally and automatically emerge when the person comes into the right relationship to him- or herself.

Living in the center of one's own authentic life experience, taking a grounded approach to life's problems, tuning in and learning to identify and address inner needs, and keeping a balanced perspective comprise the process and path to life beyond A.D.D./A.D.H.D.

In moving toward that goal of A.D.D./A.D.H.D.-free living, people with the negative symptoms of the disorder, as well as their parents, have been helped along the way by the activities, techniques, and approaches that follow.

Meditation

Meditation, as an activity, is a *natural antidote for problems of focusing and impulse control* because meditating involves quieting the mind, focusing inward, and mastering impulses. Meditation is nothing more—or less—than getting in touch with, and giving some attention to, our innermost core selves. The root word of meditation comes from the Latin word for middle—a synonym for *center*. When we meditate we seek wisdom by quieting our inner chatter and allowing the core self to be felt.

If you are reading this saying something like, "Meditate? You don't know my son (or daughter), ladies! It would be impossible for him!" our reply is to challenge you to start with yourself, learning to meditate in any way that is relaxing and pleasant for you. If you begin to take the time—even a small amount of time—to focus inward a few occasions a week, and stick with it for about two months, we predict that you will receive many benefits from your investment.

Do not try to force meditation on your child. Instead, let his or her interest and exposure grow from your own authentic experience with it.

Teaching children to meditate need not be a heavy or ponderous experience; as little as thirty seconds is long enough for a child's first encounter. As exposure increases, A.D.D./A.D.H.D. decreases.

Approach the process in the spirit of fun. For example, tell the child, "I'm going to pretend that I am floating through space in a spaceship for a few minutes, and that's all I'm going to think about," or, "I'm going to imagine that I am floating, and that's all I'm going to think about," or, "I'm going to imagine that there is a bright, warm light shining on my heart, and that's all I'm going to think about for just a minute. Do you want to do it, too?"

If you time your invitation to when your child is already more calm, we predict, based on experience, that the child will be far more receptive than you would have imagined before you began to meditate.

Natural Brain Stimulation

People who suffer from symptoms of A.D.D./A.D.H.D. require more, not less, brain stimulation. When you consider that 25% of the oxygen taken into the lungs is sent directly to the brain, and the shallow breathing pattern of most A.D.D./A.D.H.D. people, the first place to begin that stimulation is in deep, full breathing.[9] Teaching a child to breathe deeply, from the belly, will do much to keep the child's brain supplied with what it needs.

The following activities all stimulate deep breathing; finding the ones to which you or your loved one have the greatest attraction and making them a regular part of your life is an enjoyable way to move beyond A.D.D./A.D.H.D.: singing, hiking, dancing, martial arts, in-line skating, trampoline bouncing, vigorous play, sack races, running, stage fighting, calisthenics, arm wrestling, badminton, tennis, bike riding, walking the dog, hand jive, electric slide, and even the macarena. . . .

Recommended Nutrients for ADD/ADHD

The following natural substances have had a positive effect on ADD/ADHD symptomatic people. None of them are harmful in proper dosage. Check dosages with a holistic clinician.

L-Tyrosine (or Tyrosine) - This important amino acid affects mood, sleep, energy and more. Tyrosine occurs naturally in almonds, avocados, bananas, beef, dairy, eggs, fish, lima beans, pumpkin seeds, sesame seeds and soy. Tyrosine supplementation has been found to improve mental functioning and reduce stress. Begin at 50 mg., increase incrementally to 300 mg., depending on response.

Calcium/Magnesium - Use in combination, calming to nervous system, take at bedtime. Naturally occur in almonds, seeds, figs, apples, green veggies, dairy products.

Vitamin C - Supports immunity and adrenal function. Naturally occurs in fresh fruits and veggies. Safe up to 1000 mg.

B Vitamins - Regulate brain function. Naturally occur in whole grains and vegetables. Use 50mg. Vitamin B Complex. Vitamin B6 out performed Ritalin in reducing hyperactive behavior in at least one study.

Zinc and Iron - Use in combination. Calming to nervous system. Occur in pumpkin seeds, whole grains, lean meats.

EFA - Essential Fatty Acids are vital brain nutrients, often deficient in ADD/ADHD patients. Supplement daily up to 1000mg. EFAs occur naturally in cold water fish, flax oil, evening primrose oil.

Children will eat healthy food happily as long as it is served without a lecture, when the kids are hungry. Many parents have gotten good results from serving crudite and sliced fruit for snacks. Put it out without comment before dinner, don't call it "supper" and watch them eat it up!

Botanical Support for A.D.D./A.D.H.D.

Recommending herbs is beyond the scope of this book, but we can report that some proponents claim success against the negative symptoms of A.D.D./A.D.H.D. with the use of *Hypericum* (Saint-Johns-Wort), avena (green oats), Ginko Biloba, *Passiflora* (passionflower), linden flowers, chamomile, Fo-Ti, licorice (nutrifies the adrenals and soothes mucous membranes), ginseng, unprocessed oregano (not marjoram), and skullcap. Herbs can be taken in capsule form, in tea (infusions), or even eaten fresh in salads.

Traditional Chinese Medicine
In China, A.D.D./A.D.H.D. has increased with the introduction of a more consumer-oriented economy. According to traditional Chinese medical theories, hyperactivity is the result of too much heat (yang) in the liver, and a deficiency of it (yin) in the heart and spleen.

Researchers at the Shanxi College of Traditional Chinese Medicine treated a group of sixty-four hyperactive children with traditional Chinese herbs.[11] Dr. Wang Yurun created a syrup called Yizhi (wit-increasing) from several botanicals, which was found to be significantly effective for 84% of the children who took it.

According to the researchers, the syrup affected the level of neurotransmitters available in the central nervous system. They state, "traditional Chinese medicine has opened up new vistas for the treatment of hyperactivity."

Pycnogenol/Grape Seeds
Pycnogenol and grape seeds, powerful natural antioxidants, are frequently used in France for controlling the symptoms of A.D.D./A.D.H.D., and many Americans have now turned to them as an alternative and nontoxic answer to Ritalin.

Pycnogenol, which comes from pine trees, was introduced to the French by Native Americans in Canada who used it as a powerful medicine. The French have been studying and using it since, and in recent years they've discovered it to be a scavenger of free radicals, the out-of-control molecules that cause damage to the human system. Pycnogenol is capable of crossing the blood barrier to the brain to directly protect brain cells from free radicals. Pycnogenol, or grape seeds, boosts the antioxidant activity of vitamins E and C as well. In Germany it was found to be highly beneficial for the capillaries and blood circulation.

The beneficial effects of pycnogenol in capsule form, as well as its close relative, grape seeds, are thought to be a result of this enhanced circulation to the brain, as well as cell nourishment and cell protection.

The Limits of Behavior Modification

Second only to Ritalin, the most prescribed treatment for children with A.D.D./A.D.H.D. symptoms is behavior modification. Behavioral modification is a mode of therapy that uses rewards and reinforcements as its major tool.

For example, parents taking an A.D.D./A.D.H.D. child to the mall are instructed to carry a handful of poker chips along that will be meted out for specific good behavior. The chips can later be converted into rewards for the child.

Like Ritalin, behavior modification is effective in managing the negative symptoms of A.D.D./A.D.H.D. in the short run. But also like Ritalin, its effects are temporary. If behavior modification is used judiciously, as one tool of many, it can be part of a total training program that instills good habits in childhood.

However, when Behavior Modification is undertaken in a spirit of manipulation and control, the program may actually back-fire on parents or teachers who use it. That's because no one likes to feel that they are being manipulated or controlled - no adult, no teen, nor any child. At a deep level, manipulation and control result in inner resentment toward the manipulator, which may be consequently played out in passive aggression.

There may be times when you use behavior modification to manage your child's behavior. But please remember that it is best used judiciously, not as a tool of manipulation or control. Use it to simply to set a standard of behavior and the means to achievement.

Carefully select the particular "carrots and sticks" that reflect your child's stage of development. Make them appropriate and meaningful to the child for best results.

It's also essential to deliver behavior modification techniques in the spirit of offering a guideline or aid to the person's inner development. It should never be used as punishment, merely the loss of privilege. Rewards should never welcome smug self-satisfaction, but instead, leave a child with a sense of accomplishment and mastery.

10

A.D.D./A.D.H.D. in the Schools

True attention involves reasoning: it means that the child has a question of his own and is actively seeking to answer it.

John Dewey, 1915

American schools are in trouble, and everybody knows it. That educational achievement has declined is an established fact. Beyond lowered standards and achievement, problems in our school systems, particularly the public school system, are certainly clear to all who have ears to listen.

Stand quietly near any group of people discussing the schools, and you are apt to hear parents complaining about school administrators and teachers, teachers complaining about certain parents and children, and children complaining about being bored and having to go to school at all!

Into this mix comes the added factor of A.D.D./A.D.H.D. and learning-disabled children, who are walking though school doors in growing numbers. How can teachers and parents empower children to have a more valuable experience in the classroom? How can parents and teachers of A.D.D./A.D.H.D. children create the conditions that will engender a true love of learning? How can teachers empower themselves to deal with children with attention and impulsivity problems?

Creating schools that work for all children—and A.D.D./A.D.H.D. children in particular—is the focus of this chapter. If the schools work for children by helping them to become motivated to learn, we can be sure that they will work for parents and teachers, as well. This chapter offers specific, practical techniques for educators working with A.D.D. children, which are designed to foster communication and mutual support between teachers and parents.

When A.D.D./A.D.H.D. Goes to School

Symptoms of A.D.D./A.D.H.D. in school:
- School phobia
- Attention problems
- Fidgeting
- Sloppy handwriting
- Social problems with peers
- Excessive need for attention
- Daydreaming
- Inability to wait for one's turn
- Trouble copying from the board
- Impulsive blurting out of answers
- Disrupting the class in an effort to gain attention
- Work neglects detail
- Self-critical
- Auditory wipeout (child hears but does not receive information)

School Phobia

Tim

When Tim walked into Mrs. Connor's second-grade class, he brought an unseen world with him—the world of his family.

Though he was seven years old, Tim had not yet separated from his parents in a way appropriate for a child his age. Standing alone was a terrifying experience for him because he had no image of himself and little experience of himself as an independent person.

As the baby in the family, Tim was used to getting a lot of attention, most of it focused on his adorable looks and funny clowning. Tim's mother, Ruth, babied him, catering to him in the kitchen and tending to him in the bath. If Tim needed a tissue, for instance, it was Ruth who walked across the room to get it for him. If Tim had homework, Ruth planted herself next to him at the kitchen table, helping, helping, and helping. Her strength and capability as an individual seemed to be available to her only when she was playing off of a family member.

Despite her outward appearance of independence, Ruth was actually dependent and clingy inside, and she acted as if she could hardly bear to watch her sons grow older. Her role as a mother was an anchor for her in life, and she was inwardly terrified about getting older (which was represented by her children growing up and gaining independence). Instead of facing her need to create a life with interesting work or some other meaningful purpose, however, she doted on Tim and his older brother.

It followed logically that, given this situation, Tim resisted going to school. As children are prone to do, he sensed his mother's unmet need on the deepest level, and hated the idea of leaving her. By playing the part of a dependent baby, Tim was living out his mother's hidden desire: to keep him with her.

School-day mornings were filled with unpleasant feelings as Tim dawdled over his cereal, trying to delay the inevitable. When his mother finally left him at the school door, he walked in with his head low and his chin trembling. In the classroom, because his inner sense of self was insecure, he felt scared about having to stand "on his own two feet," and consequently, he looked to his teacher to fill the space his family had always filled. He treated Mrs. Connor as if she was a surrogate mother.

But the teacher could not dote on Tim the way Ruth did. She did not find his jokes amusing when they disrupted her class, and Tim's need for excessive attention became an irritant to a teacher with a large classroom.

Tim also lacked the ability to realistically assess his own skills. Because of the excessive attention and praise he had gotten at home, part of him felt grandiose and entitled to constant attention. When he didn't get it, he felt wounded and deprived. Because he didn't have enough experience of himself as a person separate from his family, he therefore had difficulty with independent thinking and felt inadequate in the classroom. These painful dynamics naturally interfered with his ability to focus on his lessons.

Tim was evaluated by the special education team in his school, and later referred to the Center, where he began doing the work that would free him of his underlying terror of being separate from his mother. As he gradually gained an image of himself as a separate entity, with thoughts, feelings, and a body all his own, Tim grew more capable of standing on his own. His negative attitudes toward school began to shift, too.

As the idea was reinforced in him that "growing up is learning to take care of yourself," *he began to sense for himself that his behavior had been inappropriate.* Following work with his root points and body ownership, he began to initiate his own process of emerging, automatically discarding the old cowering behaviors. In the past, for instance, he shrank back from contact with other boys, but now he asked to join a soccer team.

When his mother complimented Tim's therapist for her fine work with Tim, Tim piped up quickly, "She didn't do the work, Mom. *I* did. My*self*." And he was right. Tim now had a self that he was aware of, and finally he was free to "outgrow" his fear of school.

Motivating Children with A.D.D./A.D.H.D.

If the question is, "How do I motivate A.D.D./A.D.H.D. children to learn?" the answer is, "It can't be done." The far more important question to ask is, *"How do I create the conditions that will allow the children's inner motivation to emerge?"*

Ask any healthy three-year-old: learning is a joy! Figuring out, solving problems, doing puzzles, mixing solutions, sleuthing, examining closely, and wondering all come naturally when children are in the right relationship to themselves.

Beyond that, everyone has a talent; everyone is drawn like a magnet to one subject or another in all kinds of combinations. The pleasurable work of life is discovering, developing, and using those bits and pieces of talent and abilities, integrating them into a whole life's work.

Considering the natural enthusiasm and verve young children bring to learning, the current state of our schools seems especially distressing. If we are to improve our educational systems, we must first remove the obstacles that stand in the way of our children's natural desire to find out how life works. Creating the conditions that will allow the child's inborn love of learning to emerge is the true purpose of education, because *self-motivation is the only motivation that counts.* And it counts double for A.D.D./A.D.H.D. children, whose inner selves are less developed than their peers.

Teacher Empowerment

Empowerment starts with the teacher's own intention to stay centered and grounded, so that he or she can be fully conscious and present. A teacher who is self-aware and self-accepting will naturally and automatically function more effectively.

Factors That Interfere with the Natural Love of Learning

- Fear of failure—"What if I get it wrong?" "What if I fail the test?" "I'd better not make a mistake!"
- Fear of success—"What will they expect if I get it right?" "Now they'll think I know more than I know."
- Manipulation by rewards—"Reading must be pretty boring if they give you all these stickers and prizes to do it."
- Having no say in one's education—"Who cares about the Civil War, anyway?" "I don't want to learn that now." "Why do they tell us what to do, think, and feel all day long?"
- Boring lesson content—"This is the hundredth ditto like this!" "This book is too easy."
- Sitting in a chair for too long—"I wish, I wish, I wish I was outside playing!"
- Feeling invisible—"The teacher doesn't really know I exist." (This is heightened for A.D.D./A.D.H.D. children, who hardly know that they exist themselves.)

It's the process of tuning in to one's self and staying in one's own experience, *taking care of oneself on the inside*, that enables a teacher to naturally and harmoniously claim authentic and benevolent power. When the adult is personally secure and in the right relationship to him- or herself, children tend to respond with respect.

Using Group Dynamics to Create Energy Bonds

Group therapy leaders have a secret. When members first enter the space where the group is meeting, the leader will make "small talk" with every individual before calling the group together. By this process, the leader is creating an energy link with each individual, a connection that will be useful later when the group process opens up. Because of his or her personal relationship with each member, the entire group will have an invisible, but valuable, feeling of cohesion.

This energy bond is vital in classroom situations, too. It's the difference between twenty-five people thinking some version of, "Uh-oh, I'm alone with all these other people!" and those same twenty-five people feeling safe and secure, among people who know and accept them.

Creating an energy bond is most important for A.D.D./ A.D.H.D. children, who are lost inside themselves. Making sure they get a friendly greeting with full eye contact and a little personal attention when they enter the classroom each day will soothe their tendency to feel isolated and alienated in group environments.

Intragroup energy bonds, in which teachers help children to get to know one another one-on-one, are also important for a healthy classroom experience. It doesn't have to be the beginning of the year for kids to introduce themselves to one another! Try this group exercise to boost the connection of the children in your classroom:

Push the desks off to the side, making space in the middle of the room. As music plays, let the children shake out their hands and move around a little. Then, as if playing musical chairs, shut off the music and instruct the children to find a partner. Have them stand facing their partner, making eye contact, as each takes a turn telling the other what his or her favorite game is and how to play it. Have them shake hands when they are finished.

The next time you do this exercise, have them share another piece of information with a new partner. This intragroup energy bond provides an opportunity for children to be real and connected in the moment, which leads to an enhanced experience of being in the classroom.

Collaborate

Children are natural-born problem-solvers when the problem presented to them is genuine or meaningful for them. Ask the A.D.D. girl in your room what she thinks will make her experience better. How can she help herself to stay tuned?

Get input from the A.D.H.D. boy about how else he can use that energy of his without intruding on other people. Write the children's suggestions down on a card or a sticky pad. Better yet, have *them* write their suggestions down, to keep them in view during the day.

Collaborating with children gives them a working experience of how to navigate their way through the day, the week, the school year, and ultimately, life. The secret of successful collaboration in the classroom is *really needing and wanting the children's assistance in solving problems.*

At first, some children will shy away from the process of true and sincere—not made up—collaboration. These children are not used to being consulted about what works or doesn't work for them in school. But, if you sincerely want fresh and stimulating ideas, when you consult with children you will surely get them.

Some of their ideas may be impractical, but a surprising amount turn out to be rooted in good old common sense. By initiating more collaboration into the educational process, you will be giving students a say in their education. This experience of self-mastery and personal power has the lifelong benefit of enhancing self-esteem and helps youngsters to move beyond A.D.D.

Talk About It

Putting ideas that may seem obvious to us adults into words is a simple but potent way to teach A.D.D./A.D.H.D. children about the way the real world works, and how they can have a better time of it!

For instance, a common problem of A.D.D./A.D.H.D. children is that they are unaware of the difference between school and home. Asking your children to talk about that difference, and how it relates to their behavior in school (and yours, too) gives them a chance to clarify this issue for themselves.

Ask them what a student is. What's the difference between being a son or daughter and being a student? Then just listen, without any agenda. You're apt to see them come spontaneously to a better understanding of their role in the classroom.

It's amazing what direct talk with children will reveal. Put your dilemmas out there for them to think about: "There are twenty-eight kids in the class, and I want to hear what you are all thinking and feeling. But if everyone talks at once, I won't hear a thing. Do you guys have any suggestions about how everybody can get a chance to communicate? How can we manage that?"

Own Your Personal Space; Model Personal Space

Personal space is the physical area around every *body*. Personal space is every individual's personal domain. It's the territory that comes with being human. Children (and adults) with A.D.D./A.D.H.D. tend to invade other people's space and to allow others to invade theirs. They may push, pull, or cling. Those without hyperactivity tend to shrink away from purposeful activity, floating off, as if unconnected to their personal space.

Teaching an A.D.D./A.D.H.D. child the basics of body ownership is a powerful but often ignored way to help the child become anchored and grounded in space—in other words, self-possessed.

The basic message you need to get across is simple but profound: *The space around me belongs to me. The space around you belongs to you. When our spaces come together, it's got to be comfortable for both of us.* This simple message carries great impact.

Use your arms to show what you mean by personal space, by indicating an imaginary boundary around yourself with your arms. "This space belongs to me. You have space that belongs to you, too. It's the space around your body."

As a teacher, or parent of more than one child, you will have ample opportunity to teach about personal space. When one child crowds another, reinforce the concept by saying something like, "Hey, that's so-and-so's personal space. No invading allowed."

Model awareness of your own body space: "Excuse me, I need more personal space now."

Children's spaces are often invaded; by pointing out your own need for body space comfort, you teach children to assert their own need for comfort and autonomy in their personal space. Modeling healthy personal boundaries will eliminate a lot of future frustration in children, because when their space is invaded, they will know exactly what to say and do.

Make Time for Daydreaming

The uses and techniques of daydreaming are practically unlimited. In daydreams we can practice skills, expand awareness, inspire ourselves to greater achievement, and find our ability to both comfort and motivate ourselves. Daydreaming also allows us to get to know ourselves better, for in daydreams the hidden part of the mind often emerges and becomes available to us. In daydreams, teachers will find a wealth of information about children's authentic selves.

In addition, daydreaming is a wonderful tool for gaining

an experience of relaxation, which in itself opens the door to more positive life experiences and is an effective antidote for anxieties, such as math anxiety, or test-taking phobias.

Teachers who make use of daydreaming are providing their students with a direct experience of an expansive ability of the human mind. All children daydream, of course, and so do all adults, so it is all the more dismaying that daydreaming has traditionally been seen as the enemy of learning, and not the powerhouse it actually can be!

Daydreaming, visualization, guided imagery, and meditation are all closely related and can be effectively used to enhance the social and academic performance of people with A.D.D./A.D.H.D. These activities are quiet, calming, and effective. They make excellent use of children's brainpower, while giving children an opportunity to know themselves *on the inside, where it counts.*

Useful Daydreaming

Children love to daydream, and they are delighted to be given the opportunity to do it openly.

For a dramatic but calming experience, the key is *using your voice* to carry the feeling of relaxation, drama, or whatever you are exploring. Utilize the children's sensory memories, too, by mentioning as many sense-related objects as possible, such as "the bright blue sky," or "you pick up a handful of marbles; feel how smooth they are. . . ."

Following are a few basic scripts to get you started; we predict you will soon be having fun creating material of your own.

After a visualization session, it's fascinating to allow time for a discussion of the children's personal responses. When children share their daydreams, they are sharing themselves at a deep level. Listening will bring rich rewards to the teacher wise enough to use these techniques.

Daydream Scripts

Tell your students: "It's time to daydream, children." This statement will perk their interest right away! Tell them the purpose of the daydream, such as to get ready for another activity, or to relax and refresh themselves by imagining something pleasant, or to come up with creative ideas. Based on our experience, you will be a very popular teacher for using these techniques.

Continue: "You can put your head on your desk if you want to, or just sit up and get comfortable. . . . Then close your eyes and take a few deeeeeep breaths. . . . Deep and easy breaths . . . that's right . . . let yourself relax . . . and now . . ."

- For creative writing in the early grades (creative writing is an activity that promotes good brain functioning by balancing the brain hemispheres):
  ". . . imagine that you are walking by a beautiful lake . . . the air smells so fresh, and a breeze is blowing through the green leaves of the trees . . . you can see the fluffy, white clouds reflected in the water. Suddenly, you see a fish in the lake . . . but not an ordinary fish . . . it's a magical fish . . . and it can talk . . . it has a special message for you. . . . When you are ready, pick up your pencil and write about the fish . . . I wonder what your fish looks like? What makes it magical? What does the fish have to say to you? . . . write it down. . . ."

- For improved academic performance (which builds self-esteem):
  ". . . think about when you were very little; so small you didn't even know how to add one plus one. . . . But then, one day, you looked at the numbers, and you suddenly understood what adding was all about . . . and it seemed so easy after that

. . . and then you were so happy . . . you felt sooo good about yourself. . . . What was it like for you to feel that good? Can you imagine the way you felt? Now pretend you are bigger, like you are today . . . and pretend that the same thing is happening with long division. . . . You're sitting with your pencil, confused and struggling, when all of a sudden, you don't have to struggle any more . . . because you get it. . . . Imagine the look on your face, and the happy feeling inside you . . . so proud . . . you do two problems in a row, and it's not even hard . . . soon you're doing them just as you do your other work. . . . Long division is like a puzzle or a game now. . . . And solving a problem is fun—like solving a puzzle. . . ."

- For improved social skills (which strengthen secure sense of self):

    ". . . Now imagine you're outside on the playground . . . on a beautiful day, with a bright blue sky, and you're having such a great time . . . but then, a kid walks up to you . . . a kid you're a little scared of . . . and he gives you a dirty look . . . and calls you a bad name. . . . How would you feel? Some of you may feel sad; you may want to cry . . . or maybe you feel angry . . . and mad . . . I don't know how you would feel—only *you* know that. . . . Now imagine that he wants you to fight with him . . . but you decide to do something else . . . something that makes you feel good about yourself, and stops the bullying. . . . See yourself doing it. Is it something you say? . . . Would you walk away? I wonder how *you* would handle not getting into a fight?"

Allow plenty of time for sharing after the daydreaming session, with the focus on listening to what "came into" the children's minds. Children gain feelings of safety and acceptance when they can share in a nonjudgmental atmosphere, and this in turn strengthens and attunes their innermost sense of self.

Boosting the Sensory Experience at School

- Invest in a popcorn machine, and take popcorn breaks.
- Experiment with natural aromas; discuss them with the children.
- Use music as often as possible. Have it playing when they arrive; utilize it as a ritual, such as creating Mozart snack breaks every Tuesday, or jazz Wednesdays.
- Have a box of cloth (or cardboard) rectangles of many different colors and patterns. Have the children "set" their desks with the fabric of their choice before they tackle difficult work.
- Use wind chimes and bells to signal the change in class activities.
- Introduce a fruit or vegetable each day for class exploration. For example, have a few sprigs of parsley on hand one day, a few plums the next, a large cooked sweet potato, lemon, etc. Cut tiny pieces to offer tiny tastes. Allow kids to talk about their personal experience of the taste. (For more "whole learning," discuss the history, geography, nutrition, or folklore of the food item.)
- Be alert for tactile opportunities. For example, in the previous exercise, pass the food around so that each child can touch it before it gets cut up for sharing.
- Take in a bunch of grapes, and challenge the children to see how slowly they can eat just one grape.

- Be alert for opportunities to bring movement into learning. To keep any chaos down, limit the number of kids moving at any one time. "OK, anybody who is wearing red, you can take a couple minutes to walk around the room and stretch. Next the kids wearing blue will have their turn."
- Use the long view. Children are famous for looking out the window during lessons. Surprise them by setting up a "window watch"—time to gaze, observe, and notice what's going on in the outside world. (For further whole-brain learning, have them write about what they see and how they feel about it.)

The Importance of Active Learning

Think about someone who wants to teach you how to take a picture. Imagine the person standing across the room, holding up a picture of a camera cut from a magazine, as he or she tells you the basics of how it works. How interested would you be?

Now imagine that the teacher is holding a real camera and explaining it to you. You want to take a picture, but the teacher wants to talk about the camera. Might you feel a little irritated? Frustrated? Perhaps you would tune out, becoming bored?

Now imagine the teacher walking over to you and handing you the camera. Imagine the weight of the camera in your hands and the empowered feeling you get when the teacher gives it to you. The teacher is showing his or her trust in you, too, by treating you as a person who is capable of holding the camera securely. With the camera in your hands, the explanation of how it works comes to life as you learn to identify the various parts.

This example illustrates the experience of active learning, of course—in which students are participants, not audiences. Active learning is the new frontier of modern education, one of those valuable new/old ideas! Long before the advent of formal schools, active learning was how our ancestors passed on skills from one generation to the next.

Parents and teachers of all children, but particularly A.D.D./A.D.H.D. children, are well advised to hurry the process of active learning along, by advocating it as a style of learning in the schools their children attend.

To set up an active learning curriculum requires our school administrators to think and plan creatively, opening up the process of learning, taking it down from the high shelf of theory and placing it in the center of the class, where it can be touched and examined.

Active learning leads to true and lasting understanding, with results that cannot be faked, manipulated, or blown off. Experience is truly the greatest teacher—always has been, and always will be.

Practical Tips for Teachers of A.D.D./A.D.H.D. Children

- Place the child with his or her right ear closest to you, since the right hemisphere is associated with verbal learning.
- Make a couple of large placards that read, "Quiet," or "Get ready." Children with problems in sensory integration will benefit from seeing instructions in addition to hearing them.
- Use a buddy system for helping children stay on target.
- Allow A.D.D./A.D.H.D. children to set the rules as often as possible.

The Trouble with Behavior Modification

One of the most common methods of gaining control in the classroom, a method that is also a highly touted treatment therapy for A.D.D./A.D.H.D. children, is behavior modification. This popular interpretation of behavioral psychology is a system of control carried out through the use of rewards and consequences.

If you think about a circus act with seals jumping up, clapping their fins, and balancing balls, you will have a good mental picture of behavior modification in action. The seal trainer has a little pail of fish which he doles out to the hungry animals in return for their performance.

Behaviorism is popular with teachers and parents because it appears to be effective, and *is* effective in the short run. But a closer look at this increasingly common phenomenon casts doubt on its usefulness for bringing out self-motivation. It's interesting that our increasing reliance on positive reinforcements and rewards, as well as punishments and consequences, coincides with our falling national educational performances. Is this just an accident?

Going back to the seals for a moment, you notice that the show is over when the pail of fish is empty. In other words, there's no need to perform anymore when the reward is over and done with.

The seals were motivated by a force outside themselves, and so, being dependent and fairly smart, they did what they had to do to gain the reward. When the reward was finished, so was their motivation. *The same process happens to our children when we try to motivate them from the outside.*

Study after study after study has verified that rewards and incentives simply do *not* work for creating lasting learning or self-motivation.[1] The popular notion that a reward will stimulate a child's natural interest in a subject, which he or she will then pursue independently without the reward, has unfortunately been found time and again to be invalid.

For Parents: How to Handle
a Difficult or Negative Teacher

1. If your child and the teacher are having a conflict, get the teacher's side of the story and do your best to empathize with it. Teachers have a tough job; they need parental cooperation.
2. Be respectful, even if you are angry or upset with the teacher. Speak your mind, but be diplomatic in your verbal communications.
3. If the teacher tends to be boring or dull in the classroom, offer positive suggestions for more active learning, such as hands-on assignments and more collaboration with and among students. If teachers cannot offer choice in the curriculum, they can still offer choice about timing of learning and other details. Follow up on whether the teacher is using your suggestions or alternate ideas to make learning more active.
4. If the teacher tends to be destructive, belittling, or humiliating with your child, try to get your child transferred out of the class.
5. If you are stuck with an unpleasant teacher, brainstorm to help your child to come up with ways to cope with the situation. For example: "It sounds as if your teacher is pretty cranky. Maybe he's having a bad year for some reason that has nothing to do with you or your class. How can you help yourself out during the day? If you get too bored, what can you do that won't get you in trouble?"

Yes, a boy will read ten books to get a free pizza—but *don't expect him to love reading because of it.* As soon as the contest is over, the books will go away and Sega will reappear, unless the child is motivated to read *from the inside.*

Children sense when they are being manipulated, perhaps more keenly than adults do. And they are masters at playing along, working the system for all they can get. That's just their healthy self-interest in action. But if our long-term goal is to create the conditions that will allow a child's inner self-motivation to emerge, an important first step is reducing rewards and consequences.

A far better and more constructive use of our energy is exploring with each child to find out what *truly* interests the child and what the child him- or herself wishes to learn. This process of collaboration is one of the important "C" factors that lead to healthy development and solid self-esteem based on a realistic appraisal of oneself. By collaborating with our children we are helping them with the most basic developmental task of all: getting to know themselves and their potential.

When children are offered choices about their education, their inner motivation naturally rises, along with their self-esteem. Energy that has been spent resisting the educational process will then be freed for use in learning.

Active Learning

The following scenario shows what a third-grade math lesson might look like if it included active learning, choice, and collaboration.

As the children enter the classroom in the morning, their teacher, Ms. Colby, makes contact with each and every one of them, as an individual. Her greeting may be short, but she makes sure to catch each student's eyes and let them all know that she values her one-on-one relationships with each of them.

A large see-through container filled with jelly beans sits on the teacher's desk. When the children ask why it is there, Ms. Colby keeps her answer short. "Oh, that's for math."

For Teachers:
How to Handle a Negative Parent

1. Try to see the parent's point of view.
2. Assure the parent that you personally like his or her child and hope to provide the child with a positive experience.
3. If the parent is upset, hear the parent out, but remain calm and strong as you listen.
4. Remind the child of his or her autonomy.

This sets the children wondering, trying to figure out for themselves why it is there.

"Today we've got reading, social studies, and math on the agenda," the teacher announces. "How should we decide what time to do each lesson?"

"I know!" a student pipes up. "We could vote on it!"

The children vote to put math first, probably a direct result of the jelly bean jar in their midst.

"OK, guys, here's the problem: I met a big purple monster on the way to school this morning, and he said if we didn't come up with an exact count of the beans in this jar, he's going to come to school and gobble them all up, " Ms. Colby tells them. "I'm sure we all want to avoid that!" After the children enjoy the joke, she asks, "Seriously, how can we figure out exactly how many beans are in this jar?"

"How about if we take them out and count them one by one," a boy suggests.

"That would work, but it might take a long time," Ms. Colby replies.

"I know," a student calls out enthusiastically, "we could count them a few at a time!"

"Counting them a few at a time is called multiplying." The teacher's answer gives the children a chance to consider what multiplication really is. She instructs a few students to distribute *an equal share of the beans to each child, which allows them some movement.*

"OK, there are thirty-one of you, and you each have twelve beans. How are you going to find out how many there are in all?"

"We could just add 12 plus 12 plus 12 plus 12 plus 12 until we have them counted for everybody," a boy suggests.

"That would take too long," another responds.

"Hmmmm, . . ." murmurs Ms. Colby. "Well, if there were a way to get the answer in one minute or less, would you want to know it?"

"Yes!" the class eagerly responds.

"Then, I'll show you," Ms. Colby says with a smile, turning to write on the board. "We've got 12 jelly beans and 31 people. Here's what we do—"

Ms. Colby has the rapt attention of everyone in the class when she puts the problem on the board. The students are actively learning a useful skill of multiplication. When the answer comes, the jelly beans are eaten—not as a reward, but as a celebration.

(Why is this not a reward? Because getting the jelly beans is not contingent on getting the right answer, and they are never offered with conditions or strings attached.)

Only when students are fully and actively engaged of their own free will, learning material that has genuine use and interest for them, will true learning occur. This is doubly true for the A.D.D./A.D.H.D. student who is lacking a secure sense of self.

The rightful job of every teacher, and every parent, is to stimulate the child's sense of personal autonomy and independence. For teachers and parents of attention deficit-identified children, developing these qualities is all the more important; without them the A.D.D./A.D.H.D. child will be lost. The use of praise and rewards, too, must be minimized if the child is to develop a realistic sense of his or her own potential and limitations, and an authentic inner self-motivation.

Teaching A.D.D./A.D.H.D. children does not require tricks; it requires a thorough understanding of the dynamics of the disorder. The teacher must be aware that the child's internal sense of himself or herself is insecure and underdeveloped. The disorganized, frantic behavior that looks to all the world like disrespectful bravado (particularly in the case of A.D.H.D. children) is really part of a desperate attempt to flee an internal emotional environment that is intolerable. Similarly, the withdrawn and foggy behavior of the A.D.D. child is not designed to annoy teachers; it is simply the best way the child had found so far to avoid experiencing more emotional pain.

The wise teacher or parent who can see beyond these behaviors and lead children to the discovery of themselves will be helping to set a life free. Remember that we cannot learn any subject until we learn about ourselves. Only when this process is under way will our love of learning be real, lasting, and founded on our most precious inner resource—joy.

11

Building a Bridge to Recovery

When you are able to flow with and channel your energies, you will become like a sailboat that happily and effortlessly travels the rough but beautiful sea of life by using all winds including opposing ones to propel you forward. . . .

Elan Z. Neev, M.D.

In our A.D.D. world, nobody makes it to Chapter 11 in any book without having some sort of conviction about, or connection to, the ideas the book contains. Since you've stayed with us this far, we trust that you have also made a commitment to moving beyond A.D.D./A.D.H.D. in a way that is natural, holistic, and positive, as well as effective.

We trust that you are also feeling empowered by this decision, and rightly so, because making a commitment of this magnitude requires great courage. Remember that you are not alone—others have walked this path with success, and if you will do what it takes, you will move beyond A.D.D. sooner than you think.

To overcome A.D.D. in our stressful world depends on being able to practice and apply simple, natural ideas, such as staying centered and grounded and in the right relationship to yourself. For parents, it means modeling these behaviors over the long haul. *This is simple but not always easy.*

The difference between those two concepts particularly applies here. Moving beyond A.D.D./A.D.H.D. really is a simple process that unfolds moment to moment, allowing you to slowly but surely win back yourself and your loved one from A.D.D./A.D.H.D.—with no toxic side effects at all.

The results—a healthier, more authentic, expansive, and joyful life—come quickly, but they come in a two-steps-forward, one-step-back fashion, as we gain more skill in centered living and make it our own.

The task is an exciting one: to create the structures that will support your full emergence, and in the process, to provide the safety and space for your A.D.D./A.D.H.D.-diagnosed loved one to naturally and automatically discover and develop his or her own core.

As the center of your own experience, it's up to you to be alert to the messages of your higher, deeper, and truer self—the wise, all-knowing self whose quiet voice may have been drowned out by the troublesome symptoms of A.D.D./ A.D.H.D. When we are centered in our own experience, this powerful, unseen, inner self automatically points the way, lighting the path with beams of inspiration, creativity, tolerance, and love.

But like driving a car, the application of ideas such as staying centered and grounded, and being in the right relationship, requires coordination and concentration, especially in the beginning. Being fully present, centered, and grounded requires a high degree of self-awareness—one that can take us far into the world of joyful living.

Until we develop new habits of self-awareness, we may feel like new drivers who worry about keeping their hands on the wheel and foot on the gas, while being conscious of cars in the back, front, and sides of their vehicle, and do it all while switching on the headlights!

Still, if you drive, you know how driving becomes second nature. Taking care of ourselves and centering ourselves becomes second nature too, in time, but it does require some stop-and-go driving in the beginning.

We have to stop our habitual, negative-vortex patterns and go forward by focusing on our needs and creating better moments for ourselves. The welcome irony is that the more we slow down, noticing and honoring our own humanity in the moment, the faster our progress in creating positive change.

In the end, empowering ourselves to raise our consciousness moment to moment, actively sustaining ourselves in a positive reality, seeking the good within ourselves, and being heartened by the goodness in others all proceed from a simple decision.

The literal meaning of the word *decide* is "to cut away." Moving beyond A.D.D./A.D.H.D. requires our cutting away any negative energy around our ability to heal ourselves and our loved ones.

Many people will advise you that the condition of A.D.D./ A.D.H.D. is chronic and/or permanent, rooted forever in the neurological system. The larger truth, however, is that all human beings are living, changing, and growing beings. Moving beyond A.D.D. happens naturally when the stresses you've imposed upon yourself are replaced with self-support and love.

You do not need anyone's permission to start living your life the way it was meant to be lived—in a state of conscious awareness, with the power to develop and grow beyond the disorder. Let those who maintain that A.D.D./A.D.H.D. is a chronic or permanent condition hold on to the disorder. Where you are going, there will be no room for attention deficit because your interests, your pleasures—and whatever else is inside you waiting to be developed—will be getting the attention and love they need to grow.

But to get beyond A.D.D., you'll have to learn to turn your vehicle around with a pretty good three-point turn.

Hierarchy of Consciousness

Top

No A.D.D. Fully conscious, fully present, grounded, centered; positive energy emerging outward.

Middle

A.D.D. is a factor. Half focus, not fully in present moment, but somewhat aware; inner thoughts still pull attention inward.

Bottom

A.D.D. consumes life. Unfocused, tuned out, can't get it together, overwhelmed, speeded up or falling behind, missing in action, at the effect of inner needs.

Making Up for Lost Time

When the actions and interactions that have stalled the development process are removed, the natural movement toward self-sustaining development automatically begins. But in many cases, particularly with older children, the residual damage from the old patterns of A.D.D./A.D.H.D. will have left some developmental gaps that need filling.

Picture healthy development as a large wheel, or an upward-moving spiral. Our developmental needs will keep bringing us around to the same place over and over again until the need is filled and made whole.

Thinking back to the eight "C"s—the cornerstones of human development—we can more easily imagine how this developmental process works. Contact, connection, consistency, comfort, containment, collaboration, constructive activity, and commitment are all necessary for healthy development.

The child, or adult, who is in the process of moving beyond A.D.D./A.D.H.D. will naturally and automatically go back to the area that has not been fulfilled in his or her inner life. The child who has not been contained, for example, will go back to the place of needing containment. The adult who has never experienced consistency will need to establish a degree of consistent routines and rituals in his or her present-day life.

All of the "C"s are necessary for healthy development in their own way, and ultimately, each and every one has to be in operation in order to move beyond A.D.D./A.D.H.D.

Chris's Recovery

Part 1: The Bad Old Days—a Virulent Case of A.D.H.D.

Eleven-year-old Chris had been diagnosed as A.D.H.D. at the age of six after having one too many tantrums in school. The school authorities were not able to tolerate behavior with which Chris's parents, Maureen and Richard, had been unhappily living for years.

Maureen was an overly conscientious mother who had unwittingly adopted a codependent stance with Chris—a stance that shut Chris's father out of the family on an important emotional level.

Richard's response was a retreat into his new business, substituting work for true emotional connection with his family. As the years went by, these negative patterns became habitual. Maureen found herself growing more and more isolated in her relationship with Chris, as Richard found himself burying himself in work.

Trying too hard to be a good mother, Maureen worked hard, but unwisely, as she attempted to fulfill her internal idea about how a loving mom acted. Unfortunately, this notion was created in reaction to her own upbringing, and consequently, the real Chris was neglected. *Her efforts could not possibly reach her son, because they were rooted in her own inner needs, not his.*

When he was two, Maureen was startled by Chris's strong will, and instead of helping him to contain his impulses, she gave in to his demands whenever possible, in a futile attempt to "make him happy." Without meaning to harm her son in any way, Maureen nevertheless regularly invaded his space and micromanaged his life experience.

When she needed time to take care of the house, she'd let him watch TV freely, which also worked against Chris's healthy development and established a habit that was later hard to break.

When another child, Megan, came along, four-year-old Chris was severely jealous. He'd sometimes knock his sister off her trike and then run away laughing. Or he'd mock Megan, or verbally abuse her by calling her names. Maureen inadvertently put up with this behavior, feeling too weakened by her own stresses to set firm limits.

Maureen was relieved by the diagnosis of A.D.H.D. because she felt that it explained her son's negative behavior. She began focusing on Chris's perceived disability, and ascribed his poor impulse control and distractibility to an unseen brain disorder. Chris was put on stimulant medication despite his father's objections.

With stimulant medication and a strong behavioral therapy program at school, Chris began to function somewhat better there, but he continued acting negatively at home. By the age of nine, he had learned that he could control his mother's emotions and cause disruption in his parent's relationship—neither of which made him feel good about himself deep inside.

Chris became both sneaky and defiant, provoking his parents, especially his father, into using bad language in the process, or hitting. This in turn led to family screaming matches, with Maureen criticizing Richard for being too harsh, Chris yelling at his parents, Megan withdrawing into a fantasy world, and Maureen bursting into tears of frustration.

Chris was not expected to help around the house, nor even expected to sit at the dinner table if he didn't want to. On a material level, he had insatiable wants, but no matter how much he was given he kept wanting more.

As a result, Maureen's internal resentment about what she perceived as her "giving and giving" and his "taking and taking" became stuck and frozen. She often viewed Chris as an ungrateful and lazy child. Though she boiled with anger when others accused her son of being spoiled, it became harder and harder to avoid making that assessment herself.

The A.D.D./A.D.H.D. diagnosis became a kind of defense of Chris's irresponsible behavior; her involvement in A.D.D. organizations became a fort behind which she hid.

And so the negative cycle that had been set into motion when Richard and Maureen began neglecting their inner needs continued spinning out of control, with Maureen and Richard providing more toys, clothes, treats, and rewards than were necessary, and Chris pushing the limits of their tolerance.

Maureen's frustration and resentment would grow until she "let off steam" by saying and doing things that would later make her feel ashamed and guilty. What kind of mother, she'd ask herself in her darkest moments, tells her child that he's a loser and a jerk, as she had done in the heat of frustration? What kind of mother pours cold water onto a child's face to wake him as she had once done?

The entire family was now caught in the self-perpetuating negative vortex: the parents blaming each other for Chris's condition, Maureen idealizing Chris and refusing to see his negative behavior for what it was, both parents indulging Chris in order to stave off the intolerable feelings of losing his love or facing his ire, and Megan excessively escaping all of the problems by plugging in to Mario Brothers.

Chris thought of himself as a bad kid, deep inside. Richard avoided interacting with Chris. As if that all weren't bad enough, Maureen and Richard continued to neglect their marital relationship. Everyone in the family was miserable to the bone.

This pattern was shattered when eleven-year-old Chris was picked up by the police for throwing rocks through a neighbor's window while the neighbor was away, even though he had taken Ritalin that day. That event was the crisis that finally led the family to seek help.

Chris's Symptoms Before Recovery

- Overexcitable
- Aggressive, especially toward his younger sibling
- Fearful of going to bed at night
- Few friends
- Sneaky
- "Lazy" about chores
- Demanding and controlling
- Constantly seeking more toys and money
- Disrespectful of teachers
- Low self-esteem

Part 2: How Chris Found His Way Back to Health

Our work together shattered these negative patterns by putting the focus back where it belonged: on the authentic needs of each individual in the family. Maureen and Richard were tired of living in misery, and they quickly embraced the concepts of self-centering and starting the recovery process by looking within.

Each member of the family was urged to start tuning in to his or her self first, by discovering what he or she personally needed in order to feel safe and have a better time in the family.

In this light, it became apparent to both parents that they needed to strengthen their relationship as a couple. After some self-searching, Maureen decided that her involvement in the A.D.D./A.D.H.D. organization was actually draining her energy and robbing her of precious time to enjoy herself. When we made a list of potential pleasures for her, to her surprise, the first thing that came up was horseback riding— an activity in which she had not participated since she was in her teens!

Scheduling an afternoon of riding just once a month was not prohibitively expensive and gave her something of her own to which to look forward. Maureen and Richard also "redesigned" their transitional times, particularly the time between work and home, so that when they arrived home they would be refreshed enough and ready to focus on parenting.

Maureen learned to tune into herself with deep breathing and big-muscle stretching before she arrived home; for Richard, the pleasure came in listening to books-on-tape in the car. By the time he walked through the door he was no longer "burned out." Instead he was tuned in to himself and ready to be "Dad."

As Richard assessed his needs as a father, he realized that he had lost parental authority, too. He informed Maureen gently but firmly that he would no longer tolerate her undercutting his authority. Together, when they were both feeling cool and calm, they decided on ways to join forces when Chris needed discipline, even if they didn't completely agree.

In the privacy of the marital relationship, they ironed out the most basic rules that they intended to establish at home, including the consequences for breaking those rules. They included themselves in these rules, too. For instance, since one rule was no hitting or cursing, they knew they would have to put a lid on their own acting out, even when they felt frustrated or rageful. Their containment of their own out-of-control behavior is a good example of how people start with themselves.

Using lists and a parent-empowerment workbook, Richard and Maureen reviewed their own childhoods so that they could clearly identify the ways they were either blindly imitating their parents or parenting in reaction to their own inadequate childhood experiences. Their awareness of these formerly hidden dynamics protected them from falling into negative patterns.

When the underlying causes of Chris's problems were understood by Richard and Maureen, they put their concentration on centering and grounding themselves, so that they would be the calm, effective parents Chris needed. They were then ready to begin building a bridge that would take them, and both their children, into the land of recovery from A.D.D.

Without burdening Chris and Megan, or giving them undue power in the family, Maureen and Richard opened a family discussion at a time when every member was calm enough to receive new ideas. To the children's surprise, they apologized for letting things get out of hand in the past, and explained that things were going to change at home. This meeting was to announce their intention to take charge of creating a better family life, and issue an invitation to the kids to join them in "helping the whole family to turn over a new leaf."

Maureen and Richard were honest and direct about telling their children that they had given them too much power in the family. In effect, they were now putting the children in their place—the children's place, with all its attendant privileges and responsibilities, while they assumed the benevolent power and authority of the parental place, with its attendant privileges and responsibilities. This open discussion surprised Chris and Megan, to say the least.

In the spirit of turning the situation around, the parents presented the children with a short list of two basic rules "to start them off." They talked about why the rule was made and what the consequence for breaking it would be.

The top of the list was "No Hitting"—which was to apply to all members of the family, even the grown-ups. They first sought the children's input about what it felt like to want to hit, and later brainstormed with the children about what they could do instead of acting out bad feelings.

Next on the list was "Respectful Communication Only." "Look, we all have to live together and that means that sometimes we're going to disagree and argue with each other, and get mad," Richard explained, "but we're not going to get anyplace if we curse or call one another names. What do you think about what I'm saying? Do I have a point?" Megan spoke up, saying that she felt bad when Chris called her a "dork." Chris in turn said he didn't like being called a "brat," an insult both parents had given Chris when they were enraged with his behavior.

The family brainstormed about what they could do the next time any of them found himself or herself boiling with anger. Together, they composed a list of helpful behaviors and posted it on the refrigerator. This list included time-honored temper controllers such as slowly counting to ten, going into another room to cool down, drawing an ugly picture, and taking a walk. Megan said she could stomp her feet, so this was added to the list, too. Maureen and Richard emphasized that anger was OK and that it absolutely needed to be expressed, but only in a respectful way.

They taught the children the simple technique of starting sentences with the word "I" in the heat of anger, so that the person could focus on his or her true experience. Maureen used an example from her own experience. "Instead of saying, 'Chris, you're so lazy! You didn't pick the towel up!' I could say, 'I'm frustrated about seeing towels on the floor.'" "If you say it like that, I won't be mad about being called lazy, and I'll probably pick them up," Chris agreed.

It was decided that cursing would be fined and that the money would be given to charity.

Maureen and Richard limited the family rules that first meeting to no hitting and respectful talk only. They kept the list to two, not because they did not want to add other rules, but rather because they did not want to overwhelm the kids with changes. They fully intended to cut back on TV and video game time (and were ultimately successful), but they wisely waited a couple of weeks to introduce these changes. *Remember, recovering from A.D.D./A.D.H.D. goes faster when we slow down!*

Chris and Megan both responded well to this initial meeting, because they felt more connected to a healthy family process. However, eleven years of A.D.D. living had taken their toll on Chris, and part of his response included a testing period which lasted for several weeks.

During this testing period, he broke the rules on several occasions, attempting to provoke his father to swat him or curse, and he himself cursed in order to see if he would really be fined. He was.

Maureen learned to ride out the storm, even when she felt shaken inside, by containing her feelings of discomfort and keeping on a steady keel, for her own sake and Chris's. When her son's money ran out, Maureen began withholding treats instead. She did this in a nonpunitive, cool, and collected manner.

If Chris cursed, she'd simply say, "The rule is Respectful Talk," with no further lecture or upset. Later, however, when they were out, if he wanted a bottle of soda pop, she'd say, "No, you may not have it because you cursed today." If Chris became furious about that, *she tolerated—but did not get involved with—his feelings.*

Over a period of weeks and months, his parents passed Chris's tests by remaining calm and centered in the face of any provocations. When Maureen was tempted to fall into the old pattern of letting Chris get away with teasing his sister, she learned to strengthen her inner resolve by talking to herself in a supportive way.

There were times when Maureen had to order Chris to go to his room. At first he refused, but when he sensed her inner conviction, backed up by a consistent, systematic loss of privileges, he learned to comply.

Maureen learned to focus on the long view when disharmonious incidents occurred at home. Previously, if there was a family upset or dispute, she would take it to heart, dramatically proclaiming her distress. When she instead put her focus on staying in the center of her own experience, she could more easily blow off the unpleasant incidents that are part of parenting. When Chris was tired one night, and made loud, unreasonable demands on his parents, for instance, she quickly put the incident in perspective and let it go. In the bad old days, she would have lain in bed worrying about Chris or feeling inadequate as a mother. Now she listened to beautiful music, concentrating on making a pleasant transition to sleep and getting off to a better start in the morning.

In the face of Chris's provocations, Richard, too, remained calm but strong. When he felt himself on the verge of saying things he'd later regret, he took responsibility for his frustration and withdrew from the discussion to cool off in private.

By remaining calm and strong, for weeks and then months, Maureen and Richard were modeling self-containment, which in turn allowed Chris to learn how to manage his own emotions. Regularly applying the same rules met Chris's need for consistency, too. The teachers at school noticed the improvement in his behavior, even at times when he was not taking Ritalin. Within six weeks his dosage was reduced; after six months, the Ritalin was phased out completely.

Creating a Safe Environment

Once they understood the process of healthy development, Richard and Maureen set about creating a safe environment in their home, one that could contain any negative impulses and allow them to connect to their own and their children's emerging core selves. They focused on establishing their home as a place with the following attributes:

- Free of criticism, fault-finding, and blame

- Each person's basic dignity is honored

- Free of yelling, hitting, and other dramatic, out-of-control behavior

- Ample physical and mental space for each person to be him- or herself

- Parents act and interact instead of *reacting*

- Free of the excessive outside influence of TV, electronic games, and other media

- Constructive, skill-building crafts and projects are readily available

Maureen's Needs

These are the authentic needs that Maureen identified for herself and how she met them:

Need to feel calm inside—Met by soothing, supportive self-talk, remembering to breathe, and taking three-minute meditation breaks

Need for adventure—Met with horseback riding, planning vacations, and day excursions

Need for safety in home—Met with firm rules of no violence and no tolerance of unsafe behavior

Need for connection with Richard—Met with plans to begin "dating" her husband on a regular basis; new exploration in sex; arranging little surprises for Richard

Need for peace and quiet at home—Met by playing soft music at times, making time to watch sunset, and staying inwardly quiet at times (starting with herself)

Need to feel special—Met by treating herself to manicures, dressing with more dramatic flair

Need to contribute to society—Met by joining Sierra Club and becoming active in environmental issues, writing letters to newspaper

Need to connect to other women—Met by reaching out to old friends and scheduling time with them, being aware of and nurturing new potential friendships

Richard's Needs

Here are Richard's authentic needs and how he met them:

Need to balance work with play—Met by limiting work hours, delegating tasks at work, and finding ways to work smarter, not harder

Need to get in better shape—Met by joining a local basketball practice group, joining the local "Y" so he could swim in winter

Need for grown-up male companionship—Met by hosting a monthly penny-ante poker game, assessing old friendships and being available for new ones

Need for greater authority at home—Met by asserting authority in a firm but benevolent manner

Need for romance—Met by reintroducing courting behaviors with Maureen

Swinging in the Hammock: True Connection

Once Chris's parents learned to center and ground themselves, and tune into their inner needs, they could connect with him in a more genuine way. They were now able to be calm and strong even in the face of childish behavior. The idealized image they formerly had of Chris no longer stood in the way of a truly connected relationship with their son. Maureen touchingly spoke of a moment that occurred just three months after she and Richard began empowering themselves to move beyond A.D.D. The moment perfectly illustrated how developmental steps that were skipped over or incomplete can be revisited.

On a summer day when Chris was twelve, he went to the hammock after supper. The table had been cleared (by Chris), but the kitchen still needed tending. Nevertheless, Maureen put the housework on hold and went outside to sit near Chris while the sun went down.

Without speaking, she met Chris's eyes and smiled. He smiled back as she sat down near the hammock. To her surprise, Chris said, "Rock me like a baby, Mom." She nodded peacefully and began gently pushing the hammock for several minutes.

"When Chris was a baby, I was usually too nervous about doing everything right to just be peaceful like that," Maureen told us. "This time I felt so calm, and he did too. We didn't even say anything, because we were both so content. A few minutes later, he got up and began playing with Megan, but I noticed he was in a good mood that whole evening."

Twelve-year-olds aren't often rocked like babies, and moments like these cannot be planned. That swing in the hammock offered an opportunity to revisit an earlier developmental place. It represented a way that Chris and his mother could heal their formerly troubled relationship.

Moving Beyond A.D.D./A.D.H.D.

To move beyond A.D.D./A.D.H.D. means moving into a state of free living, in which pleasure, friends, talents, abilities, and preferences can be explored from a balanced center, in a spirit of self-discovery. *Moving beyond A.D.D. means taking your center out into the world, opening yourself up to new experiences and adventures, and actively taking charge of and designing your life.* Only you, in your most centered place of knowing, can tell what this exploration will lead to in your life. As with sensory integration, each individual—child or adult—must determine for himself or herself how to spend the precious energy of life. We have seen formerly bedraggled, discouraged parents of A.D.D./A.D.H.D. children perk up, full of vibrancy as they rediscovered old friends, took up gardening, or started singing or playing baseball.

In that spirit of open exploration, this section briefly explores three areas that are particularly useful to people in the process of pushing past the limitations of A.D.D./A.D.H.D: connecting to nature; spirituality; and arts, crafts, and family fun.

Forging a Bond with Nature

A strong bond with nature is a powerful remedy against the condition of A.D.D./A.D.H.D. Interacting with nature, as a gardener, hiker, fisher, birder, walker, sky watcher, stargazer, boat rower, camper, and more, is highly useful in combating the symptoms of the disorder.

The slow pace of nature is the perfect opposite of the hyped-up, speeded-up, stressed-out condition of A.D.H.D. Exposure to natural places and involvement in natural processes teaches many lessons over time. It is fascinating to see A.D.H.D. children, who may be bored with the slow pace of nature at first, loosen up and come into focus in nature's splendid presence. This process is gradual, of course, and requires repeated exposure to the natural world, but we have never seen it fail.

To be in a safe, natural environment with an A.D.H.D. child, allowing him or her plenty of latitude for exploration and play, is far more powerful than many artificial remedies over time. Resonating with the pace and richness of nature is a tonic for the A.D.D./A.D.H.D. psyche.

For both A.D.D. and A.D.H.D. individuals, repeated experiences in outdoor activities such as camping, rowing, swimming, and gardening promote self-mastery, which in turn combats low self-esteem. Learning the skills needed to participate in the great outdoors is a proven confidence builder.

Observing wildlife, too, forces the A.D.H.D. child to gain patience and slow down to a natural pace. For A.D.D. children who have a hard time attending to details, wildlife observation is likewise beneficial, as it builds focus and persistence.

Time playing and exploring nature also promotes sensory integration as long as we adults can stay out of our children's experience. If you can get to a place where your eyes can go far and look wide, be sure to go there: taking the long view is as beneficial for our souls as it is for our eyes.

While in a natural setting, instead of pointing out what you see so that the child has to turn to look, follow the child quietly and notice what he or she is discovering! (This technique is helpful in other places, too, even malls.)

If you are an A.D.D./A.D.H.D. parent or adult, this principle still relates. The trick is to keep the vigilant, busy mind in the "off" position and to let your spirit roam free in the natural place, opening up to the healing power of nature.

Spirituality

The *human spirit* is a term that all of us, no matter what our religion, can understand. By human spirit, and spirituality, we are referring to an energy level of being that goes very deep and very high in a human being. Spirituality is the unseen energy that connects us to the mystery and majesty of the universe. True spirituality is far from a superficial practice of religion that can be subverted and co-opted by the judging mind and turned into shallow ritual or a game of who has dibs on The Truth.

True spirituality is the living relationship between an individual and the power of the universe as that person understands it. Like any relationship, true spirituality has to be cultivated through practices such as meditation, prayer, and coming together with others to explore our highest aspirations and deepest values.

Many children are initially intrigued by spiritual practices, such as prayer, but soon put off by adult rigidity or hypocrisy in this area. We believe that revitalizing the desire to believe, however one understands that term, and putting beliefs into action, however small, are powerful weapons against A.D.D./A.D.H.D. and other conditions of imbalance. The principle of starting with ourselves applies, of course. Forcing spirituality doesn't work any better than forcing other things. But adding words of "thanks" before a good dinner, or saying a quick good-night prayer, over time reinforces the ability to believe in something larger than human life and strengthens the A.D.D./A.D.H.D. person's spiritual grounding and moral foundation.

One of the best-kept secrets in America has been the number of scientific studies undertaken at prestigious universities, notably Harvard, that prove the effectiveness of spiritual practices against all kinds of human illnesses and ailments.[1] Occasionally, one sees publicity about such a study in the mass media, but it is usually served up quickly and soon forgotten despite its profound implications. Based on these studies, we believe that paying attention to spirituality and nurturing ourselves and our loved ones with prayer is a powerful tool for healing attention deficit.

In science, the gold standard of research is the double-blind, control-group study. For example, a large group of people with a particular symptom will be assembled. Half of the group will be given a drug, and the other half will be given a harmless placebo, such as a sugar or starch pill that is manufactured to look identical to the substance being tested. The "double-blind" part means that neither the person dispensing the drug nor the person taking the drug will be aware of which tablet is the placebo and which is the substance being tested.

Dozens of such studies point to the efficacy of prayer and other spiritual practices in combating a variety of ailments. In one study, for instance, coronary-care patients who were prayed for by strangers (who had no more information than a first name of the patient) needed only one quarter of the antibiotics as the unprayed-for group. They also needed less pain relief and had shorter hospital stays—all this despite the fact that the patients did not know that they were being prayed for!

So, if you are intrigued, or inclined, consider praying for the A.D.D./A.D.H.D. individual in your life. Prayer will help you to organize your inner power and strengthen your intention to remain calm and strong as a parent.

> *Lord help me not to do for my children*
> *what they can do for themselves.*
>
> *Help me not to give them*
> *what they can earn for themselves.*
>
> *Help me not to tell them*
> *what they can find out for themselves.*
>
> *Help me to help my children*
> *stand on their own two feet*
> *and grow into responsible, disciplined adults.*

The prayer on the previous page was composed by Marian Wright Edelman, the world-renowned champion of children's causes. We include it because it so eloquently expresses a helpful point of view for parents of people with symptoms of A.D.D./A.D.H.D.

Arts, Crafts, and Fun

Boredom is a constant complaint of many American children, and most notably a problem in A.D.D./A.D.H.D. children, who require *more* stimulation, *not less*, for their development. The problem is that most boredom busters in our society are passive, such as watching TV or going to movies. Even video games provide little active involvement, only the eyes, mind, and hands are involved, and usually in an imaginary but destructive way, shooting and blasting.

Very little skill building and self-mastery go on in front of a video screen, and these, not praise, are the building blocks of healthy self-esteem. Passive electronic entertainment doesn't do much to engage a child's mind or feelings. A screen, after all, is an object that stands between us and real life.

For a family moving beyond A.D.D./A.D.H.D. plenty of hands-on activities are a must. Developing interests around arts and crafts, and keeping wide open to having family fun, are essential. We don't know how you, or your child, like to have fun, because fun has to grow from the inside out, but being alert to its possibilities is vital.

Games such as checkers, cards, board games, miniature golf, puzzles, and team sports all build patience and social skills. Reading together as a family, even when the children are older, is a wonderful way to slow down the pace of life, while providing nourishment for the mind.

Viewing a movie together and then talking about it in a way that allows everyone's opinion builds family cohesiveness and contributes to feelings of connection. When the initial shock of No Weekday TV sets in, the family may feel unsettled, but within a matter of weeks, our families report the emergence of all kinds of new creative activities, and fun. From bowling to bocci, marbles to Pictionary, family creativity and fun helps pave the way beyond A.D.D./A.D.H.D.

The Road to Recovery

When we began this book, we talked about traveling down the same road, each of us in charge of his or her own car. Using the ideas we have presented, and opening up to your own healing power and creativity, you are facing forward, your eyes steady on the road ahead, as you leave the land of A.D.D./A.D.H.D.

By choosing a holistic approach to moving beyond A.D.D./A.D.H.D., you are heading off in the direction of real life. The journey began the moment you decided to start with yourself and get out of your own way. The A.D.D./A.D.H.D. person in your life may still be standing in the way of his or her personal vehicle, but based on our experience he or she will soon be moving forward. As you persist in living fully, taking charge of your own experience, on the lookout for your needs, and treating yourself well on the inside, the A.D.D./A.D.H.D. person in your life will naturally shift his or her position, too.

For some families, change is quick, dramatic, and lasting. For others it is gradual, dramatic, and lasting.

We hope you have already started the process by taking the time to tune in to yourself and organize your life around your needs and pleasure. When you honor your internal life, create rituals and routines that nurture you, and look to yourself as the center of your experience, any blurred boundaries with others will naturally clear up, too, and you will naturally and automatically cease invading others' spaces.

Fully grounded, with your feet firm, your eyes upon the glittering stars, you can confidently move forward to a healthier future—a future filled with the development of potential—free and clear of A.D.D.

12

Moving Your Family Beyond ADD

Powerful Tools and Techniques For Parents

As a parent, you have many powers to help move your child beyond attention deficits. That's because your words, actions, and attitudes create a powerful training environment. Your household is the platform for your child's development, built of guidelines, schedules, rules, routines and rituals that *you* establish. As a parent, you have the power to encourage certain habits and behaviors, or nip destructive ones in the bud. The positive behaviors you instill and negative ones that you discourage will benefit your child long after he or she is grown.

Using your parental powers wisely, however, requires that you be secure and lovingly in charge, first of yourself, then of the household. Naturally, as an adult you have far greater knowledge and awareness of the big picture of what is truly important in life than your child has. In fact, your child relies upon you for safety, guidance, and wise perspective – even though he or she is not always aware of that reliance.

It follows that the more secure you are in your own *loving authority*, the more your child will come to trust your judgments and therefore accept the limits you set. (He or she will usually dislike those limits, but so be it. Limits are an important part of life.)

Your sense of parental power – or lack of it - comes across in everything you say and do. It is communicated by the way that you regard yourself and others. It shows in the way you communicate, how you take care of yourself, and how you handle mistakes and adversity. Your voice, your laugh, your inner strength, the attitude and manner you have toward others – all form a powerful example for the young person in your life.

So forget lecturing – there's absolutely no power in it. Instead look to *the quality of your own inner life.* Learning to maintain a confident, positive life stance will show power that will help strengthen your child for what lies ahead, and move the whole family to higher ground.

This chapter highlights tools, techniques, exercises and suggestions designed to strengthen your parental power. Only an empowered, alert and positive parent can move beyond the behaviors, mindset and attitudes of ADD/ADHD, into the light of balanced, aware, symptom-free, joyful living.

Shape Your Inner Attitudes

The thoughts we have inside ourselves have a powerful effect on our parenting. Try holding onto these healthy inner ideas throughout the day. Memorize and repeat these positive, supportive thoughts and remind yourself of them until they become second nature.

I KEEP MY COOL
No matter *what* is going on, you can train yourself to stay centered in yourself, and *not* react to a child's negative, immature behavior. Training yourself to keep *cool under fire* takes discipline that is well worth the effort. When you are centered, you will deal with problems from a higher perspective. From a position of "cool" you will naturally take a better stand and communicate with more wisdom. That's a lot better than automatically reacting, or saying something negative that you may come to regret. Best of all, your child will sense power in your restraint, and respect you for it in time.

I AM CONSISTENT

Inconsistency makes children anxious. Conversely, consistency builds security. Stop negotiating every little thing with your child. *Make few rules but enforce them consistently.* If name-calling is against the house rules, for instance, avoid giggling when your child calls someone a clever name, no matter how cute it may be. Your rules need to be updated as your children grow, but they should always be delivered consistently to build security.

MY PRIMARY RELATIONSHIP IS WITH MY PARTNER

It's easy for parents to get "hooked" into an intense one-on-one dependency relationship with their kids, especially the first child. But remember, *your job as a parent is to prepare your child for life without you.* Your child is not your life-partner; your spouse is. Keeping your adult relationship in tip-top shape will benefit the entire family, including your child.

I TAKE TIME FOR MYSELF

If you are not in the right relationship to yourself, you simply cannot be an effective parent. Children are like special magical mirrors that can see what we parents can't see in ourselves. They "reflect" our unconscious state of being. A mother who is unconsciously self-critical will have a child who points out her flaws. A dad who is always tired will have a child who gets stuck easily. *Making time to nurture yourself gives you the power to grow in positive relationship to your self, your spouse and your children.*

I PLAN AHEAD FOR EACH DAY

When we have a road map, we get where we want to go with the least amount of time and hassle. Planning is critical for everyone, and the small investment of time that it takes will be rewarded a hundredfold. Planning keeps us out of the fog and leaves us ready for timely, present moment action. Without planning, (ex. "We put out our clothes the night before school and work") we run into chaos, hurry and stress. Get in the habit of mapping out a family schedule, and stick to it!

I PAUSE TO CENTER MYSELF BEFORE REACTING

It's hard living with immature people, and during the course of a typical day many things happen that require on the spot parental responses and decisions. The calmer, more centered, and consistent our reactions at those times, the more effective we will be as parents. It helps to draw in a deep breath and physically take a step backward, away from the fray. Make sure your feet are firmly on the ground and then respond. Your parental instincts will kick in and you will know when to use a firm or gentle tone, or how to pull a child aside for private correction. Being in control of your words and actions is the first, critical step.

I KEEP A JOURNAL or SKETCHBOOK

Self-expression has multiple benefits for parents (and kids.) You can vent in a journal, or figure our new solutions for thorny problems. You can draw your feelings, or write supportive letters to yourself, filled with encouragement. You can write a funny poem about family life that shifts your attitude. Journals and sketchbooks help us to validate our own experiences and keep them in perspective.

I LOVE MY CHILD JUST AS S/HE IS NOW

Children take any critical comments or judgments very personally, way down deep in their cores. Your child's sense of self grows and develops based on the "gleam in your eye." Be ready with a smile when your child comes home from school. Separate your child as a unique and wonderful human being aside from any problem areas. Your child's behavior, attitude, and ability to organize may need improvement, but he or she is really "A"-OKAY - an absolutely beautiful, perfect, uniquely wonderful human being – AS IS.

I HUG MY CHILD DAILY

The daily hug is a powerful demonstration of loving connection between child and parent, valuable from toddler to teenage years and beyond. Your physical warmth and demonstration of positive feelings is *critical* for proper human development. Hugs smooth the rocky road to maturity, too. Be sure to give and receive them everyday.

I REMEMBER TO BREATHE DEEPLY SEVERAL TIMES A DAY

What a great habit to get into! Practice, practice, practice and the benefits will amaze you. Breathing through the nose, deeply and slowly is one of the very most important actions that we human beings can do to keep us calm, cool and collected. Close your eyes and breathe deeply. Feel your breath all the way down to your feet. Feel your connection to the ground fully. Need an instant vacation? Close your eyes, breathe deeply and imagine or remember being in the most beautiful place possible. It works!

I CHOOSE TO SEE THE LONG VIEW

Preparing children for adulthood is the whole point of parenting. How many years will it be before your children are legal adults? Not many! Will your child be prepared for adult life, with all its challenges, ups and downs? They will if you keep your attention on the direction of time and consciously do the work of training them - with all the love and humor you have - for the inevitable challenges that lie ahead.

Releasing the Patterns of Past Generations

No person is perfect; no family is perfect. Every family has specific patterns - attitudes, energies, ways of organizing and connecting - that pass down from generation to generation, for good and ill. How you were parented determines how you parent. Moving beyond ADD means creating a healthier family by disconnecting from any negative patterns that were instilled in you early on, by your family of origin.

No one aspires to be negative, self-critical, perfectionistic, full of complaints or always needing to be "right." Those tendencies are often the result of the dreariness and baggage of generations coming down upon us. For the sake of our happiness, it's up to us to get out from under that junk by first facing our negative shadows. Only then can we begin living our own unique, authentic, joyful, and satisfying lives.

Facing shadows takes courage and extra work, however, because we usually can't see the negative, passed-down traits in ourselves! They are simply too close to see. It's like trying to look at your spine or the tip of your nose! Nevertheless, before we create something better, we simply must rid ourselves of these unwanted traits!

Free Yourself of Family Dysfunction (Unhappiness)

These exercises are about gaining awareness of the particular negative traits that influenced *you* when you were too little to defend against them. It's not about blaming your parents and grandparents – they probably did the best they knew how. And even if they didn't, their negative influence will only be over and done with when you free yourself in the here and now!

Turn a piece of paper sideways and draw 4 circles along the top, for your grandparents. Midway on the page, make 2 circles, for your parents. Then draw 1 circle for yourself. Do one page for your family and have your parenting partner do one for him or herself.

Mark each circle with the relative's initial. Colored pencils enhance the exercise by making attitudes and traits even more visible.

Choose the emotional traits, behaviors and attitudes from the following list and write them near each person's circle. Then reflect and connect the dots: Which of these traits affected *you* as a child? How? Note the treasure that has been passed on to you as well as the trash you may have 'inherited' from past generations. How are these positions being passed down to your children?

GENUINELY POSITIVE HAPPY ENTHUSIATIC FUN-LOVING   CREATIVE   WARM   KIND   TOLERANT FLEXIBLE COMMUNICATIVE COURAGEOUS GOOD

WITH CHILDREN   CONFIDENT   BALANCED
WHOLESOME   FULFILLED   MADE   GOOD EYE
CONTACT   PLEASANT   RESPECTFUL VOICE

NEGATIVE   UNHAPPY   CRITICAL   COLD
UNFULFILLED WORRIED OBSESSIVE INTOLERANT
LONG-SUFFERING   NON-COMMUNICATIVE
PERFECTIONISTIC   AFRAID   ALCOHOLIC   SELF-
LOATHING RIGID UNBALANCED CLINGY CRANKY
AVOIDED EYE CONTACT   YELLING   SULKY

Remember, whatever you don't like that you "inherited" from past generations can go! Keep the treasure and throw out the trash!

Cut the Strings

Now that you have boosted your awareness of the negative 'strings' that have influenced your development, it's time to symbolically 'cut' them.

Stand tall, with your shoulders as far apart as possible, your feet rooted on the floor, your knees slightly bent, your head held high. Begin breathing slowly and deeply from your nose bringing air into your body, into your physical center (right under the belly button.) Your position should be strong but relaxed.

With eyes closed, reflect for a moment on each of your grandparents and parents. One by one, silently thank them for everything they passed on to you – even the difficult stuff because it helped you to learn! But now you will be 'cutting the strings' and freeing yourself of the past.

With eyes open, make your fingers into imaginary scissors and begin 'cutting' the influences of the past away from you. As you cut you can verbalize your reflections, Ex. "Grandpa, I love the way you could fix things, but I am cutting your cranky attitude out of my life!" "Mom, I appreciate what you did for me, but I am letting go of your anxiety and fear - right now!"

When you have 'cut all the strings,' lift your arms high in a position of celebration. Then let you arms open widely and symbolically receive a new flow of fresh life energy. Move your arms freely in a 'dance' of celebration. End with a giant hug of appreciation for yourself and your new-found freedom!

Take A Self Inventory

This is simple stuff - but so important! Be honest and you will soon identify the areas that need some extra energy and attention in your life.

YES or NO

I start with myself before asking others to make changes.

I silently encourage myself.

I make time for me.

I have created an interesting, fulfilling life for myself.

I am in charge of my food intake and have healthy eating habits.

I do something to boost my heart rate, a minimum of 3 times a week.

I stay in shape, mentally and physically.

I speak to others respectfully, even when I'm annoyed or upset.

Happiness is my highest goal.

I value and appreciate myself.

I can say "No" comfortably.

I have a hobby or interest other than my family.

I go out by myself a couple times a month.

I keep in touch with friends.

I prepare myself for each day.

Take a Parenting Partners Inventory

Ah, love... You meet and join forces, becoming a couple. But when children come along, suddenly you and your partner have to expand your roles to become Mom and Dad. Seldom do we sit down and figure out our parenting philosophy so that we can consciously create good guidelines to enhance our roles as parenting partners. Here's a chance to see how you and your spouse fare as co-parents. Any NO will need to be turned into a YES!

YES or NO

We make time for each other.

We have a 'date' at least twice a month.

As parents, we are "united at the helm".

We discuss discipline strategies privately before acting.

We do not put each other down, especially in front of the children.

We settle disagreements privately.

We discuss our visions and dreams for ourselves and our children regularly.

When we have a problem we discuss it openly and respectfully.

Take a Parent Inventory

Okay, be brave! Here's a short parent inventory that will show you how you are doing as a parent.

YES or NO

I express unconditional love for my child every single day.

When I am feeling critical or annoyed by my child, I keep my cool.

I set limits on TV and video game use.

There's more healthy food in our house than unhealthy food.

When I am feeling critical, I stay silent and handle the problem inside myself.

I give my child space and encouragement to solve his or her own problems.

I offer positive perspectives to my child.

I am careful not to over- praise.

I give my child enough "space" to be him or herself.

I supply my child with the kinds of experiences that will help him or her to stand on his own two feet.

Establishing Routines and Rituals

It's comforting to know what we have to do, how to approach it, and to repeat an action until it becomes a routine. Routines enable us to follow through in life without having to reinvent the wheel or become emotional. A positive routine allows you to "go on automatic," doing what you need to do, as you build your life day by day.

Here are typical routine times that you probably face during the school year:

- Getting up
- Getting out of the house
- Homework
- Mealtimes
- School nights
- Bedtime

Take some time to think about these activities and how they occur over and over on a daily basis – for several years. Go over each of the times in your mind. How can you create the smoothest, most pleasant routine for it?

Consult with your children to get their opinions and input about each possible routine. When they are invested in creating the routine, they will take more initiative.

Get creative. Maybe there's always a plate of fruit on the table during homework time. Maybe you ring a bell to signal when the kitchen is "open" at dinnertime. Maybe you play certain music during breakfast and at bedtime.

Remember parents, you have the power to set rules for these routine times, too. Ex. "No TV on school nights." "Bedtime is 8:30." The consistency you establish will help your children feel secure deep inside, (no matter how they complain!)

Sure, there will be bumps and exceptions, but the better you establish routines in the first place, the more smoothly your family life will go.

Creating Rituals

Like routines, rituals create a comfortable frame for our lives. Try creating fun rituals that match your child's growing maturity: Family forum, family game night, Saturday morning pancakes, bowling or hiking on weekends, the same special dinner to celebrate academic achievement, Earth Day litter pick-ups and picnics, Christmas in July, or a special Appreciation Day for each family member. Celebrate half-birthdays, put a good luck object in a person's shoe before they go off to a new place, have kids write what they're grateful for on Thanksgiving and keep the papers to read through the years.

Repeated rituals enhance and improve your family experience in ways that will live on in memory long after your children are grown.

Establish a Family Forum

A family forum keeps the members of a household well-organized and positively connected. Meetings should be short, fun, and useful. Choose a time and day when the family will meet and stick to it to form a habit. You can meet around a table or sit in a circle on the floor. (Note from Avery: I used to put a small chocolate 'kiss' at each member's place, and this helped get the kids to the meeting!)

Start with a short summation of the good things that happened in the past week. This is the time to highlight new skills learned or positive behavior.

Then move onto open communication, when family members can make requests, or discuss problems. Ex. "Now you can talk about anything you want. If something is bothering you, this is the time to let us know so we can understand. We may not be able to help, but we will try." Use an egg timer to limit, and avoid commenting during each person's turn.

It helps to have a symbolic object handy, like a special stone or stick. The rule is that when a member has possession of the object they have the floor. No one is to interrupt or interfere, and others are to listen respectfully. This technique is drawn from the Native American tradition.

When the adults connect and center their energies on having a well run meeting, the family will begin to move in a harmonious, cooperative direction. Make sure everyone has enough physical space around themselves. Ignore minor infractions unless they are truly heinous. For example, if one child begins talking during another's time, don't verbally correct them. Instead stay silent and focused as you put a finger to your lips for the child who is interrupting. The goal is progress, not perfection.

Other topics to cover will be chores, events, and goals. Get creative about assigning chores. Some families write them on slips of paper and put them in a jar for choosing. Allow your children to identify solutions for getting the work done. Remember, this is not about having a free staff to clean the house; it's about training kids to pitch in, and be helpful. Start small and build on success.

Have a calendar ready to mark up-coming events. Note what each person needs to prepare for the events. This is a time to offer support. Ex. "Is there anyway that we can help you prepare for your math test?"

Lastly, use the object to go around have each person sum up his or her goal(s) for the upcoming week.

End with a special ceremonial hand-shake – ex. one fist on top of another in the center of the group, and a special 'family cheer' – Ex. Who is the best family in whole, entire universe including Mars and Jupiter? The Johnson Family! Yay!

Family Forum

You'll need: a clock or bell, a calendar, a special object, pencil and paper to write down goals.

- Sample Family Forum Agenda
- Welcome each member
- Discuss new skills learned and point out positive behavior
- Open Communication – Each person gets
- Divvy up chores
- Up-coming events
- Create goals
- Ceremonial family handshake or song

Tune Into Music

Music is a fabulous tool for creating a healthy "atmosphere" in your home. Use music for different purposes and to help your family move along in life. Music has been proven to influence learning, motivation, and focus. The vibrations of music work in mysterious ways to improve our lives, but the results are indisputable.

To engender FOCUS (ex. for homework time) offer your child a choice of music in a major key, with a steady beat about 60 per minute, simple 4/4 rhythm, no lyrics, sounds familiar, and has constant volume. (Avoid unfamiliar sounds, heavy bass, distracting lyrics.) Ex. New World Symphony, 2nd Movement, or The Great Gate of Kiev, Masursky Pictures at a Museum.

To engender CALM (Ex. Before bed) play slow, simple music, with even, flowing rhythms, continuous (uninterrupted) sound, soft to moderate volume, low pitch. Ex. Canyon Trilogy by Native American flute player, R. Carlos Nakkai (the best ever for calm)

End the Sibling Wars

Oh, no! They're fighting again, and out goes the calm from your home! First, understand that most sibling fights are unconsciously designed to gain your attention, because the kids are bored but don't know how to fill their time. Team up with them to plan ahead by making a list of cool stuff to do.

When ADD symptoms enter the picture, you have to be extra careful too. Please avoid assuming that your ADD/ADHD symptomatic child is the 'troublemaker' during sibling squabbles. Avoid protecting either child from having to take responsibility for their actions. In general, unless they are killing each other, stay out of the fray. You have the right to separate them. If they refuse, as long as they are safe, wash your hands of the situation.

Carrots and Sticks

There's no use arguing with a child - *ever*. If you find yourself in an argument with your child, you can bet that you have given up your power. Instead of arguing, have a plan to encourage better behavior.

Carrots' are rewards or perks. 'Sticks' needn't be horrible. A lot of real learning comes from the manner in which you express your disapproval. Mean it. Be firm. But don't be mean or critical.

Mom and Dad's Big Sticks
"Speak softly, but carry a big stick!"

- Toddlers: Time Out (3 minutes), take a toy away, no treat
- School Kids: Time out (15 minutes), toy taken away, loss of privilege/treats
- Pre-teens: Grounding, loss of privilege/money
- Teenagers: Ride refusal, loss of phone privileges
- Older Teens: No funds

Twenty Messages for Kids with ADD/ADHD Symptoms:

1. There's nothing wrong with you.
2. There's nothing wrong with you.
3. There's nothing wrong with you.
4. Nobody's perfect – not me, not you.
5. You have inner power that can help you be the best you can be.
6. Your inner power is with you all the time.
7. You can use your inner power to take charge of yourself.
8. You can use your inner power to make things easy.
9. When you are upset, take a big deep breath.
10. When you are mad, say why you're mad.
11. You can choose how you act in school and at home.
12. You can choose to make good things happen.
13. You can use your inner power to have fun and do better work.
14. You can figure out how to do homework without hassles.
15. You can help your family and be good to yourself.
16. Growing up is learning to take care of yourself.
17. Growing up is getting to know yourself, like a friend.
18. In a few years, you will be grown up.
19. Everything goes better when you use your inner powers.
20. There is nothing wrong with you.

Afterword

When A.D.D./A.D.H.D. is gone, a lot of negative energy goes with it! Gone are the all-too-frequent feelings of inadequacy, enmeshment, and shame. Gone are the storms and tantrums, the harangues that mark the emotional climate around active A.D.D./A.D.H.D. Gone are the intolerable feelings of frustration, fear, and daily experience of personal failure.

In the place of all that negativity is a human being—a unique human being in the process of creating him- or herself. Moving beyond A.D.D./A.D.H.D. takes us back to our creative centers, the place of true and lasting self-possession. From that center, everything good becomes possible, and everything positive can proceed.

Freed from the negative symptoms, the person can now focus on creative living and the pursuit of life's most important pleasures—making and keeping friends, developing talents and interests, and exploring the world, inside and out.

There's a kind of magic in the process of recovering from A.D.D./A.D.H.D., but no magic wand. While recovery will come naturally to anyone courageous enough to start with him- or herself, the moment-to-moment work of recovery requires patience, vigilance, and persistence.

For the adult with A.D.D./A.D.H.D., the journey to full recovery means reclaiming his or her authenticity on a moment-to-moment basis, connecting to his or her inner self, honoring that self, and living comfortably within the body. The new action of touching base with oneself, opening up the senses and deepening the breath, allows the old life to heal as the new life is revealed—a life truly worth living.

Parents of A.D.D./A.D.H.D. children who embark on the journey we have explored in this book need not fear that because people can only reclaim their lives for themselves, their A.D.D.-symptomatic children will be left with the disorder permanently. As parents courageously start with themselves, they will soon begin—automatically and naturally—to create conditions that allow for the emergence of their child's authentic inner self, too.

The formerly stressed-out, confused, or discouraged parent, when living in the center of his or her own experience, fully grounded and embodied, now resonates a deep and joyful truth with his or her life—a truth that lies beneath the level of words. Such parents are powerful, living examples of how a self-possessed, tuned-in person lives.

By being securely in their own space—their parent place—and honoring their inner selves, parents will naturally deliver new and useful messages about what is expected, and what will be tolerated. And because they are actively meeting their own needs, they do it from a place of calm, supportive, loving kindness.

The person who has the courage to start with himself or herself becomes like a glowing lamplight—a warm light that shines in the darkness of A.D.D., allowing others, too, to find their way out.

No pill or medication will ever transform the symptoms of attention deficit. On the contrary, an outside medication for this human dilemma of A.D.D. will serve only as yet another symbol of personal defect, robbing valuable self-confidence and wasting precious time that would more usefully be spent facing the issues that stand in the way of self-development.

Instead of investing hopes in chemical agents with no proven efficacy, the person who moves beyond A.D.D./A.D.H.D. will turn his or her attention to living from a growing center, nurturing him- or herself on the inside, where it counts. The business of life, once this process is started, becomes advancing to our own potential, enjoying ourselves and our loved ones as we go.

In the continued presence of adults who are authentically rooted in themselves, even children with the worst symptoms of A.D.D. will emerge from the negative effects of the disorder.

They begin to discover their natural interests and inclinations and move to developing them. Their reputations with others slowly but surely begin to be restored as they re-form themselves from the inside out, and automatically gain social skills rooted in self-respect and respect for others. In time, they will mature into responsible teenagers and young adults who move forward in life with a purpose that is rooted and alive, deep within themselves.

We've seen it. We've been there. And we can say with assurance that it happens as naturally as plants grow toward the sun. If you have taken advantage of the information and ideas in this book, and let them sink deep into your consciousness, you already have had an experience of this process within yourself. And you have probably already discovered, as we continue to discover, that the "hard" work of recovery is actually easier and lighter than the old, out-of-kilter way of living. Grounding oneself at the very core, taking charge of one's life, tuning in to oneself in an accepting, friendly, and supportive way is what real life—joyful life—is all about.

Yes, there is a transition time as old habits die and new ones emerge. Yes, we need to do the work, sorting out ourselves from others and letting go of old baggage. Of course we must take charge of our negative habits, re-form our commitments, and remind ourselves to stay on center. But what a reward awaits people who are willing to empower themselves to live! When we get out of our own way, our energy rises, and we can truly move toward fulfillment with joy.

There's not a person on this planet who cannot make the shift we have described in this book. Laying down the symptoms of the disorder is more than possible—it is necessary. A.D.D./A.D.H.D. destroys happiness, and therefore, it has no place inside the human heart. From this moment forward, pull yourself back to center by acknowledging your true inner needs and set yourself free.

We are grateful that you have walked this path with us. Please know that we are out there, too, doing the work within ourselves. One by one, we can free ourselves. Together, we can shift our society and infuse it with our humanity. But we will accomplish this good only by starting with ourselves, at center, living in our body home, by taking charge of ourselves and taking full responsibility toward our experiences. Only then will we be able to lovingly connect to everything that is valuable and real in life. Only then will we be free to be ourselves, allowing others to be themselves, and moving forward together in the joyful dance of life beyond A.D.D./A.D.H.D.

Notes

Introduction

1. Wallis, Claudia, "Life in Overdrive," *Time*, July 18, 1994, 43.

2. Biederman, J., Faraone, S. V., Mick, E., Spencer, T., Wilens, T., Kiely, K., Guite, J., Ablons, J. S., Reed, E., and Warburton, R., "High Risk for Attention Deficit Disorder Among Children of Parents with Childhood Onset of the Disorder, a Pilot Study," *American Journal of Psychiatry*, 1995, 152: 431-35.

3. See Wallis, note 1.

4. Colborn, T., Dumanski, D., and Meyers, J. P., *Our Stolen Future* (New York: Dutton, 1996), 193.

5. Mander, Jerry, *In the Absence of the Sacred* (San Francisco: Sierra Club Books, 1991), 83.

6. Hallowell, Edward M., and Ratey, John H., *Driven to Distraction* (New York: Simon and Schuster, 1995), 12-13.

7. Kohn, Alfie, "Suffer the Restless Children," *Atlantic Monthly*, November 1989, 98.

8. Deutsch, G., Papnicolaou, A. C., Bourbon, W. T., and Eisenberg, H. M., "Cerebral Blood Flow Evidence of Right Frontal Activation in Attention Demanding Tasks," *International Journal of Neuroscience*, 1987, 36, no. 1-2: 23-28.

9. Malone, M., Kershner, J. R., and Swanson, J. M., "Hemispheric Processing in ADHD," *Journal of Child Neurology*, 1994, 9, no. 2: 181–89.

10. For more about brain activity, see Michael Hutchinson, *Megabrain* (New York: Ballantine, 1991).

11. "Psychotherapy Found to Alter Brain Chemistry," *New York Times*, November 15, 1994, Section B.

12. Moyers, Bill, "Healing and the Mind," Public Broadcasting Service, 1993.

13. Micheal Meaney of McGill University found that stressful versus stimulating experience actually "altered both the receptors for certain brain chemicals and the gene for the receptors." Sociologist Dorothy Nelkin of New York University argues that the notion of an all-powerful genetics—able to cure and explain personality—is appealing because "it lets you blame everything on the individual's biology. If nothing is the result of social forces, it grants society a certain absolution."

14. Ibid.

15. See Biederman, note 2.

16. "Diagnosis and Treatment of Attention Deficit Disorder in Two General Hospitals," Walter Reed Hospital Army Institute of Research, July 1989. This study also found that only 19% of families were involved in psychotherapy and only 16% had a school intervention plan. The overall quality of care was found to be inadequate in more than two-thirds of the A.D.D./A.D.H.D. cases studied.

17. Jensen, P. S., Xenakis, H., Shervette, R. E., III, Bain, M. W., and Davis, H., "Diagnosis and Treatment of Attention Deficit Disorder in Two General Hospital Clinics," Department of Military Psychiatry, Walter Reed Army Institute of Research, 1989. In the world of mental health,

A.D.D./A.D.H.D. symptoms are often linked with depression, anxiety, and post-traumatic stress, which also cause inattentive behavior and personal confusion. Several studies indicate that children with the disorder have significantly more impaired cognitive, family, school, and psychosocial functioning than controls. Other medical and dietary factors that resemble A.D.D./A.D.H.D. include hypoglycemia, nutrient (particularly mineral) deficiency, and thyroid disorders. Thyroid disorders affect approximately 5% of people with A.D.H.D.

Chapter 6

1. Castleman, Michael, *Nature's Cures* (Emaus, PA: Rodale Press, 1996), 32–42.

2. Steele, J., "Brain Research and Essential Oils," *Aromatherapy Quarterly* 3 (1984): 5.

3. Franchomme, P., "Aromatherapy on the Wards: Lavender Beats Benzodiazepines," *Journal of Aromatherapy* 1, no. 2 (1988):1.

4. See Castleman, note 1.

Chapter 7

1. William Reich, Ida Rolf, Moshe Feldenkrais, Mattius Alexander, and Meir Schneider are a few of the luminaries who focused on the body as a way to open, explore, and expand the self and to correct any emotional, mental, or psychological discomfort energy blocks.

Chapter 8

1. Mander, Jerry, *In the Absence of the Sacred* (San Francisco: Sierra Club Books, 1991), 83.

2. Goleman, Daniel, "How Viewers Grow Addicted to Television," *New York Times*, 1991, Section C, 18.

3. Ibid.

4. Ibid.

5. Ibid.

6. Murray, M., and Pizzorno, P., *Encyclopedia of Natural Medicine* (Rocklin, CA: Prima) 372–76.

7. Rappoport, J. L., "Diet and Hyperactivity," *Nutrition Review*, 44 suppl. (May 1986): 158–62.

8. Egger, J., et al., "Controlled Trial of Oligoantigenic Treatment in the Hyperkinetic Syndrome," *Lancet* 1, no. 8428 (March 1985): 540–45.

9. Harley, J. P., et al., "Hyperkinesis and Food Additives; Testing the Feingold Hypothesis," *Pediatrics* 61, no. 6 (1978): 818–28; N. Feingold, *Why Your Child Is Hyperactive* (Random House, 1975); Rowe, K., Hopkins, I., and Lynch, B., "Artificial Food Colourings and Hyperkinesis," *Australians Paediatric Journal* 15, (1979): 202; Lipton, M., and Mayo, J., "Diet and Hyperkinesis, an Update," *Journal of the American Dietetic Association* 83 (1983): 132–34.

   The largest study of the Feingold diet occurred between 1979–1983, when over 800 New York City schools used the diet. Despite the fact that only lunches were involved, the rise in overall student performance was dramatic. See Schoenthaler, Stephen, et al. "The Impact of Low Food Additive and Sucrose Diet in Academic Performance in 803 New York City Public Schools," *International Journal of Biosocial Research* 8, no. 2 (1986): 185–95.

   Research that discredited the Feingold diet was underwritten by the Nutrition Foundation, an organization funded by the makers of Coca-Cola, Fruit Loops, C & H Sugar, and other junk-food manufacturers. These studies, though widely publicized, were largely discredited by the scientific community. See Swanson, J., et al., "Food Dyes Impair Performance of Hyperactive Children," *Science* 207 (1980): 1485.

The Feingold Association of the United States can be reached at P.O. Box 6550, Alexandria, VA 22306.

10. "Culture of Addiction," radio documentary hosted by Kilian Ganly, March 1996, WBAI-NYC, Pacific Radio.

11. Ibid.

Chapter 9

1. Breggin, Peter, "Insight on the News," *Washington Times*, August 14, 1995.

2. "Hyperactivity," *All Things Considered*, National Public Radio, airdate July 13, 1995.

3. See *New York Times*, note 1.

4. Kolata, Gina, "Boom in Ritalin Sales Raises Ethical Issues," *New York Times*, May 15, 1996, Section C, 8.

5. Klein, R. G. F., "Clinical Efficacy of Methylphenidate in Children and Adolescents," Columbia University, College of Physicians and Surgeons, Encephale (March–April 1993): 89–93. See also *Physician's Desk Reference*, 49th edition, 1995.

6. A closer look indicates that 9% of children treated with methylphenidate developed tics or dyskinesias (other involuntary motor impairments) of which 1% went on to develop Tourette's syndrome. See Lipkin, P. H., et al., "Tics and Dyskinesias Associated with Stimulant Treatment in Attention Deficit Disorder," Long Island Jewish Medical Center, *Archives of Pediatric Adolescent Medicine* (August 1994): 859-61.

7. "Does Ritalin Cause Cancer?" *New York Times*, January 13, 1995.

8. Nasrallan, Henry, "Cortical Atrophy in Young Adults with a History of Hyperactivity," *Psychiatric Research*, 1986, 245.

9. Swami Rama and Balantine, Rudolph, *Science of Breath* (Honesdale, PA: Himalayan International Institute of Yoga Science and Philosophy of the U.S.A., 1979): 30–31.

10. *Journal of Biological Psychiatry*, 1979, as cited by Autism Research Institute (formerly Child Behavior Research Institute), June 1992.

11. Yuanling, Sun, "Clinical Observation and Treatment of Hyperkinesia in Children by Traditional Chinese Medicine," *Journal of Traditional Chinese Medicine* 14, no. 2 (1994): 105–09.

Chapter 10

1. For a fuller discussion of the dynamics involved in intrinsic, as opposed to external, motivation, we highly recommend the following two books: *Punished by Rewards*, by Alfie Kohn (Houghton-Mifflin, 1993), and *Why We Do What We Do*, by Edward I. Deci (Grosset Putnam, 1995).

Chapter 11

1. For a more complete discussion of this issue, see the work of Dr. Larry Dossey.

Bibliography

Armstrong, Thomas. *The Myth of the A.D.D. Child.* Dutton, 1995.

Ayres, Jean. *Sensory Integration and the Child.* Western Psychological Services, 1995.

Ballantine, R., S. Rama, and A. Hymes. *Science of Breath.* Himalayan Institute of Yoga Science, 1979.

Breggin, Peter. *Toxic Psychiatry.* St. Martin's Press, 1991.

Breggin, Peter, and Ginger Ross Breggin. *Talking Back to Prozac.* St. Martin's Press, 1994.

Brennan, Richard. *The Alexander Technique Workbook.* Element Books, 1992.

Castleman, Michael. *Nature's Cures.* Rodale Press, 1996.

Deci, Edward L. *Why We Do What We Do.* Grosset Putnam, 1995.

Diamond, John. *Your Body Doesn't Lie.* Warner Books, 1979.

Faber, Adele, Mazlish and Elaine. *How to Talk So Kids Will Listen and How to Listen So Kids Will Talk.* Avon, 1980.

Faber, Adele, and Elaine Mazlish. *Your Guide to a Happier Family.* Avon, 1990.

Hallowell, Edward, and John Ratey. *Driven to Distraction.* Simon and Schuster, 1994.

Holt, John. *How Children Fail.* Dell, 1964.

Hutchinson, Michael. *Mega Brain.* William Morrow, 1991.

Igram, Cass. *Self-Test Nutrition Guide.* Knowledge House, 1994. (To order, (800) 295-3737.)

Keleman, Stanley. *Embodying Experience.* Center Press, 1979.

Keleman, Stanley. *Patterns of Distress*. Center Press, 1989.

Kohn, Alfie. *Punished by Rewards*. Houghton-Mifflin, 1993.

Lott, Lynn, and Intner, Riki. *The Family That Works Together*. Prima Press, 1995.

Lowen, Alexander. *The Language of the Body*. MacMillan, 1971.

Mander, Jerry. *In the Absence of the Sacred*. Sierra Club Books, 1991.

Murray, Michael, and Joseph Pizzorno. *Encyclopedia of Natural Medicine*. Prima Publishing, 1993.

Norden, Michael. *Beyond Prozac*. HarperCollins, 1995.

Robbins, John, *Reclaiming Our Health*. H J Kramer, 1996.

Rozman, Deborah. *Meditations for Children*. Aslan, 1989.

Russell, Peter. *The Brain Book*. E. P. Dutton, 1979.

Schneider, Meir. *Self-Healing*. Arkana, 1989.

Stewart, Mary, and Kathy Philips, *Yoga for Children*. Simon and Schuster, 1992.

Index

3

Similar books by
Transpersonal
☀ Publishing

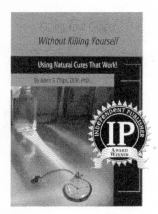

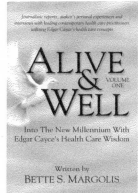

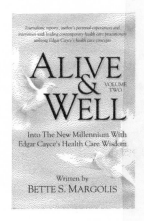

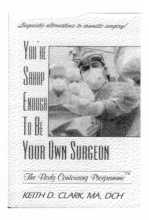

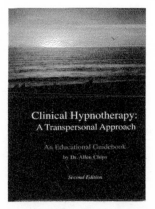

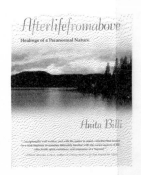

www.TranspersonalPublishing.com